NOT DEAD YET

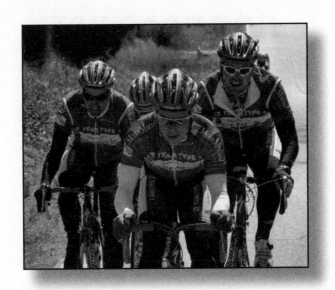

PHIL SOUTHERLAND and JOHN HANC

NOT
DEAD
YET

MY RACE AGAINST DISEASE:

FROM DIAGNOSIS TO DOMINANCE

Thomas Dunne Books

St. Martin's Press ≋ New York

THOMAS DUNNE BOOKS.
An imprint of St. Martin's Press.

NOT DEAD YET. Copyright © 2011 by Phil Southerland and John Hanc. All rights re-
served. Printed in the United States of America. For information, address St. Martin's
Press, 175 Fifth Avenue, New York, N.Y. 10010.

www.thomasdunnebooks.com

www.stmartins.com

Library of Congress Cataloging-in-Publication Data

Southerland, Phil, 1982–
     Not dead yet : my race against disease: from diagnosis to dominance /
Phil Southerland and John Hanc. — 1st ed.
          p. cm.
     ISBN 978-0-312-61023-4 (hardback)
     1. Southerland, Phil, 1982—Health.   2. Diabetic athletes—Florida—
Biography.   3. Cyclists—Florida—Biography.   4. Diabetics—Family
relationships.   I. Hanc, John.   II. Title.
     RC660.4.S636 2011

First Edition: May 2011

10   9   8   7   6   5   4   3   2   1

To my mom, Joanna,
my brother, Jack,
and every mother and father out there
trying to raise a healthy child

Contents

Acknowledgments

Acknowledgments from Phil and John

This book would not have been possible without some special people whose contributions we would like to recognize:

Our agent Linda Konner for her wise counsel; our editor Pete Wolverton for his support, encouragement and his superb editing; Anne Bensson for her efficiency and organization; and bike racer-writer Kathryn Bertine, for her special contributions to this book, which Phil and John greatly appreciate.

A very special thanks to Phil's friends and family, who gave so generously of their time, memories and insights to John: Chris, Joe and Dave Eldridge, Ray, Daniel, Andy, "Father" Phil, Jack, Kevin, Dr. Wright, Vassili, David, Sheila and, above all, Phil's remarkable mom, Joanna . . . our heartfelt thanks.

In addition, each of us have some people to acknowledge:

Phil Would Like to Thank

My author, John Hanc, who has been great to work with and is someone I will consider a friend for many years to come. I don't think my story could have been told any better.

My family and my friends, who have been on this journey with me, deserve special thanks for their contributions to my life and to Team Type 1: In addition to my family—Joanna, Jack, Phil—I want to thank (and in some cases thank again!) Sheila, John, Rybo, Linda, Tom, Zak, Jerome, W.J., Michael Scholl, Bill, Kevin, Holly, Benny, Big Worm, Kent, Joe, Ed, Vee, Nathan, Ray, Louie, Jeff A., Ace, Bill Henry, Matt Winston, James Epperson, Bub Brill, Micah, Dave Crowe, John Wilson, Dr. Bruce Bode, Nancy Wright, Larry Deeb, Mike Kipniss, everyone at Camp Kudzu, Holly Kulp, Karmeen, Abbott Diabetes Care, Howard Z., Steve Bubrick, Rob Campbell, Shashank Deshpande, Khosrow Fouzouni, Kevin Buckle, Shawna, Pierre, Dennis, Michele, Esin, Frank, Vassili, Janna, Sergey, Mike C., Celina, Hank, Wes, Matt, Colby, John, Tom, Marco, and a special thanks to to all the people at Sanofi-Aventis, who are continuing to help make this dream come true, and all the passionate people who work in the world of diabetes to make our lives better.

John Would Like to Thank

Pat Capra of Lunar Sports Group and good friend Liz Neporent for the introductions; my family and friends—especially my wife, Donna, as always, my ally and sounding board; my fifteen-year-old son, Andrew, who seemed to find Phil Southerland's story far more interesting than much of what his dad is always droning on about; and my buddy Ray Sullivan, whose extensive knowledge of bikes and bike racing often came in handy. My colleagues and the administration at the New York Institute of Technology have always been supportive of my writing, and for that I thank them. I'd also like to thank Dave Berger at Gone Racing; Fred Boethling and his colleagues at the Race Across America; and the folks at the Athens Twilight Classic for providing me with information and materials on their respective events and Phil's involvement in them.

Preface

When I was seventeen years old, I confidently predicted to my kid brother Jack that I would someday start an organization that would help people with diabetes; and that it would grow to be something really big. I had no real idea of what I meant or how that would happen. I just knew I wanted to do something to fight the disease that, even at that tender age, had already been a part of my life for longer than I could remember.

You see, I was diagnosed with type 1 at seven months of age. Seven months. At the time, I was the youngest child—anywhere—known to have been diagnosed with what was then referred to as "juvenile diabetes."

Part of this book is the story of how that seven-month-old—whose mother was told that he would probably be blind, and quite likely not even be alive, by age twenty-five—has exceeded expectations and then some (I'm now 29, and I can read the eye chart just fine, thank you).

It's also about how the prediction that I made to Jack grew into something real: Team Type 1—which started with me on a bike riding from Athens, Georgia, to my home in Tallahassee, Florida and grew to the point where, as I write this now, I am on a plane flying back from Africa, where we delivered 40,000 test strips, 400 blood sugar meters, insulin, and much more to diabetic children in Rwanda.

The story of how I got there is part of this book, as well. It's also a story about a kid who grew up in a single parent home, in the New-Old South of the 1990s. And about how that kid fell in love with bike racing and dreamed of someday making it to the Tour de France, and how that dream would materialize—although not in ways he had envisioned.

When the idea of this book was first suggested to me, I hesitated. "Who am I to write a memoir when I'm still in my twenties? Lebron James?" But I realized that with all due respect to Lebron, I have also overcome a lot in my life; been through some harrowing and remarkable adventures, and have plenty to say about it. And I hope that what I have to say—put into words with the help of my writer, John Hanc—will not only interest but inspire you. Particularly if you're a diabetic, but even if you're someone facing another kind of obstacle or challenge; or if you are someone who was told they can't do or can't be something—which is something I've been hearing all my life, too.

I'd like to think that perhaps my story will help enable your story to unfold; your dreams and your plans to become reality.

Remember, they said I wouldn't even live to be twenty-five. And here I am. Not dead yet.

—*Phil Southerland, Atlanta, Georgia, December 2010*

NOT DEAD YET

Introduction

Perseverance is not a long race; it is many
short races one after another.
—WALTER ELLIOTT, *The Spiritual Life*

Athens has run amok.

The lush boughs of the city's ancient ginkgo trees are awash in garish floodlights. The grand antebellum mansions—the former residences of Confederate generals and southern textile barons—are being invaded again, this time by an army of students, the young men in their uniforms of knee-length shorts, T-shirts, and backward baseball caps, the girls in halter tops and immodest sundresses. Down stately old streets where once Stephen Foster melodies echoed, the percussive chords and shrieking vocals of AC/DC—"*Yeah,* you ... *shook me allll night lonnggg*"—now reverberate off the genteel porticoes and sidewalks.

This is Athens, Georgia, generally considered one of the most civilized burgs in the Old South; it's a university town, an intellectual and creative center. But on this warm spring Saturday, forty thousand people are packed into six square blocks, many of them spilling into and out of the forty bars and twenty restaurants that line the narrow streets of the city center. They seem anything but civilized and more intent on turning staid old downtown Athens into a scene out of MTV's *Spring Break* for one crazy night.

I'm about to ride a bicycle into the midst of it all.

My helmet is off, but my hands are squeezing the handlebars as I wait, trying to avoid having a plate of pasta and roast vegetables accidentally dumped on me by some corporate vice president's tipsy wife or husband. I'm straddling my bike in a roped-off area of VIPs, set up on the corner of Clayton Street and College Avenue. The streets are closed off today to automobile traffic in order to let my kind of vehicles hit the pavement, as this is the starting line of one of the greatest bicycle races in America, the Athens Twilight Criterium—part pep rally, part Mardi Gras, part sporting spectacle.

This is a place and a race I know well.

All day long, people on two and, in some cases, three wheels have been blasting around these streets, in a series of competitions for all ages and ability levels. They've competed on racing bikes, road bikes, hand cycles, and wheelchairs.

All day long, other people have been watching them, cheering and consuming enough beer to fill the Oconee River.

All day long, the rest of the country has been seeing Athens on its TV screens. Not because of the Twilight—it's one of the great *under*reported sports events in America, in my opinion—but because on this night, April 25, 2009, a breaking news story from Athens (a place from which breaking news rarely emanates) is just now being broadcast on CNN and FOX. Earlier today, a professor in the marketing department at the University of Georgia allegedly walked into a community-theater rehearsal in Athens and shot his estranged wife, a man presumed to be her boyfriend, and another person. A nationwide manhunt was now on for this guy. The really creepy thing is that, when I saw his face flash up on the

2

screen of the TV in my hotel room, I remembered him. While I was at the University of Georgia I had worked part-time in the marketing department, where I was studying. I recall making photocopies for this very same professor who had now allegedly murdered three people in cold blood.

One thing about us southerners, though. Tragedy and violence may be as much a part of our heritage as grits and kudzu, but we don't let anything stop us from having a good time. Unless you'd heard the radio or seen the news reports on TV, you wouldn't have known that a murderer was on the loose, possibly even in the crowd, on this boisterous and celebratory night in Athens. Since a crazed killer wasn't stopping thousands of UGA students from wanting to have a good time, see a great race, and drink a bunch of beers, it sure wasn't going to stop me and about 150 of my fellow pro riders from providing the entertainment.

Bike races in the United States tend not to attract large crowds— that is something of an understatement—but the Twilight is a striking exception to that rule. They draw big here, because they know how to put on a show. And there are few shows in all of sports better than a criterium. It's a race held on a closed loop course; basically, like NASCAR on two wheels, except that instead of blasting around a track in the bottom of the bowl of a stadium with spectators looking down, we're racing here around the narrow streets of a nineteenth-century city center, separated from the fans only by some flimsy plastic fencing.

It's a race run in circles, and they've been going in circles in Athens since this morning: kids, amateur riders, wheelchair competitors, local studs and now, us pros, who will soon race around the one-kilometer downtown course eighty times; a total of about fifty miles.

The crowd in the VIP area swirls around me and the other pro riders, who are lined up like paratroopers on a transport plane, waiting for the red light and the call to "Jump!" one by one. I've got my trusty Orbea Opal—the bike made especially for me and my team. It's a seven-thousand-dollar super-tough but superlight racing bike: The frame weighs only two pounds five ounces. The 2009 model is "completely redesigned," as they say on the Web site, "to withstand the rigors of North American–style bike racing." (I wonder what that means at Twilight . . . perhaps that my bike is beer-proof? . . . but then I realize this is not the North, as far as I'm concerned, but the sunny South). I love my Orbea, even though the company put a somewhat comical picture of me on their Web site, holding my Opal with a forced scowl that makes me look like some spandex-clad mob hit man. *(Gimme da money you owe Rocco, or I'll roll over ya toes with my skinny tires.)*

In reality, I still don't look that much different from the fifteen-year-old punk who first showed up at Twilight in 1997 sporting a Mohawk haircut and a "screw you" attitude. I would go on to compete eight times there over the years. But before I was a Mohawked teenager or a professional bike racer and team owner, I was a miracle in progress. A miracle because at that time I was one of the youngest children ever diagnosed with type 1 diabetes: seven months old when I was diagnosed. That day in Tallahassee Memorial Hospital—seared into my mom's memory so that she can still recount almost minute by minute, as if she had a video camera behind her eyes, capturing every awful detail—was supposed to have been one of my last, but with every passing day I defied both the odds and the doctors' grim predictions.

They said I would be blind and maybe deceased by age twenty-five.

By the time you're reading this, I'll be twenty-nine.

While the reports of my death were premature, the life that I lead is in many ways not all that different from the reality faced by 25 million other Americans who also live with diabetes. Imagine if you had to check your heart rate or blood pressure twenty times a day. Imagine knowing that if, for some reason, those levels changed, you could suddenly fall unconscious on a crowded city street, behind the wheel of your car, or off a bike on a lonely country road. Imagine having to make sure you carried around with you at all times the diagnostic equipment and drugs needed to prevent such things from happening, and that everyone around you was trained and prepared to inject or force-feed you some life-saving medicine in case you did pass out. Imagine a life where taking conscious, deliberate actions to stay that way is, well . . . a way of life, the focus of much of your day.

Welcome to *my* life.

Consider: the first thing I do when I wake up every morning is draw blood—my own. It's a pinprick, to be sure, but a daily reminder for diabetics that there is something inside them that always has the potential to go haywire. For the diabetic athlete, that's just the beginning. Carbs are measured like degrees in a ship's boiler room: too few, we go cold, too many, we explode. Eating is sometimes about as pleasurable as adjusting the thermostat in your living room. Meanwhile, we have to dole out the precise amounts of rapid-acting insulin that keep us alive and in balance, while monitoring the heartbeats that we endurance athletes need to keep at a certain rate to make sure we're pushing ourselves hard enough, but not so hard that we're going to black out at the top of that category 1 hill we're climbing. Numbers and units, units and numbers: I throw around terms and measurements such as basal rate, dex 4, grams, and bolus units the way baseball players use at-bats, Ks, and RBIs. Sometimes I can't even get a good night's sleep without being haunted by these numbers, a constant reminder that I'm not a "normal" person; that my life is held aloft in the very small space between a few digits that determine the level of insulin my body is producing; that, in some ways, the days are as fragile and heart-pounding now as they were when I was seven months old in Tallahassee Memorial.

Yet, I have survived. I have succeeded.

I have help. From my friends, my teammates, my physicians, the drugs that I take—and I take a lot of them. Indeed, I'm one of the few professional athletes in the world, certainly in the cycling world, who takes drugs legally, and with a clear conscience. Have to. These aren't performance-enhancing drugs; these are life-sustaining drugs.

The logos of two of them are on my jersey. Lantus and Apidra. With good reason, *beyond* the fact that the company that makes them—the French pharmaceutical giant Sanofi-Aventis—paid to put them there!

Quick lesson in diabetes: Insulin is the hormone needed to transport glucose (sugar) from the blood into the cells of the body for energy. Most people's bodies manufacture and utilize their own. Diabetics don't, so we have to take insulin; and the timing of when we introduce it into our system is critical. Lantus is long-acting or "basal" insulin, meaning that I take it once a day; it's released into the bloodstream at a relatively constant rate for twenty-four hours. Apidra is rapid-acting insulin that I take before or after a meal, to help keep my blood sugar levels from "popping." Put it this way: if I sat on my butt all day, the long-acting insulin, released into my bloodstream at a steady rate, would be fine and my blood sugar would stay where it's supposed to. But of course that's not how you should live your life. You need a second insulin that's ready to react to the "pops"—fluctuations up or down—that occur when you eat or exercise. In essence, that's the yin and yang of diabetes management, right there: food raises your blood sugar, insulin lowers it. For a diabetic, it's a constant question of balancing the two. If I may say so, I've gotten good, damn good, at striking that balance. If my blood sugar is trending up, I'll take the fast-acting insulin *before* I eat, because I know that eating is going to raise it further, so I want the sugar-lowering insulin there to cover that. If it's trending down, then I'll do the insulin *after* I've eaten, so that again my levels are back where they should be. It's like trying to anticipate your metabolism's next move. There's this quote attributed to former NHL superstar Wayne Gretzky: "A good hockey player plays where the puck is. A great hockey player plays where the puck is going to be." Same here. I don't react to where my blood sugar is at any given moment; I try to manage the combination of food and insulin in anticipation of where my blood sugar is likely to be a few minutes from now.

Drugs like this have sustained us well—and the proof is in what we've been able to achieve.

In 2006 and 2007, my team—Team Type 1—won the Race Across America, aka RAAM, the legendary three-thousand-mile cross-country race that is ranked as one of the toughest endurance challenges on the planet; it's right up there with ultramarathons in the desert and U.S. Army Ranger competitions, where they jump out of planes and hike fifty miles with one-hundred-pound backpacks. Bike-racing purists find RAAM bizarre; ordinary people find it riveting. With due respect to the purists, the people are right on this one: RAAM is an incredibly tough and exciting event that captures the imagination and spirit of endurance athletics. I'm proud as hell that my team won it.

I'm particularly proud because of how far I'd come to get to that point. I remember how I felt when I led the team for the last leg of the race in 2007. We were the winners—the first cyclists to cross the finish line in New Jersey, having started in California less than five days earlier. We set a new record for riding from sea to shining sea, and every one of us was a type 1 diabetic.

The following year, we formally created a professional men's cycling team that included four riders with type 1 diabetes (I being one of them). The squad earned forty-five wins and boasted two riders who competed for their respective nations in the Olympic Games. Already in this 2009 racing season, Team Type 1 was showing the bicycling world what we could do in more-traditional team races. By the evening of the Twilight Criterium in April, we had already competed in the Tour of California, riding right next to Lance Armstrong and his team.

Lance, of course, beat his life-threatening disease. While I will probably never be able to say that I'm diabetes-free or that I beat type 1, I am living proof that diabetes *can* be beaten into submission, which is what I'm doing every day of my life, and what I try to show others how to do.

It's also the reason I'm writing this book.

Because beyond my job as the guy in charge of Team Type 1, I still have a job as the guy in charge of my type 1. I am the CEO of my body. That's something important for diabetics to understand, particularly young diabetics who feel like they have little control over anything in their lives. Well, they can exert an enormous amount of control over the disease that has seemingly taken over their lives. They may not be able to get rid of it, but they can show it who's boss by doing the things they need to: checking their blood sugar more regularly, monitoring their A1c levels, getting more exercise, eating better.

I've been the CEO of Team Type 1 since its inception in 2005. I've been the CEO of my body since I was about six years old—although tonight, as I await the start of the Twilight Criterium, I realize that my authority over that body is being challenged. Not by the diabetes, either, but by a serious leg injury that is threatening to knock me off the bike—permanently.

I look around, trying to take my mind off that. There are familiar faces here and in the crowd on the other side of the fence. Old friends from my UGA days. Amateur riders I've met at races over the years. Fans of our team whose pictures I recognize from Facebook posts on our Web site. Uh-oh. Here comes a very familiar face: my mom. I feel my jaw tightening. She's the last person I want to see right now. Before you shake your head at me in disapproval, thinking I'm some kind of bad son, let me assure you that I love and respect Joanna Southerland very much. It is only through my mom's determination, pluck, and character that I survived what I went through as a child. She was my advocate, my protector, my rescuer. She still is—even when I really don't want her to be. I know, I know . . . that's what moms do. But she's coming right up to me now with her big smile, and that camera. More pictures! Please, Mom. Even our Web site, which can probably hold ten gazillion gigabytes of photos, cannot possibly handle one more image of me.

"C'mon," she says, seeing my sour expression at her approach. "Smile!"

The truth is, my mom makes me a little nervous before races. I don't need that. I'm already amped up on Starbucks, Red Bull, AC/DC, and the Kings of Leon (who I was blasting on my iPod earlier), not to mention the nervousness that comes with being both a player on the team and the team owner. Yes, I admit it: I've been a bit cranky, a bit short with people, and probably shorter with her than anyone else. I could blame it on my blood sugar—on the fact that my daily life reads like a problem in a chemistry final, filled as if is with units of this and grams of that, all carefully measured or consumed. But to say that I'm cranky because of my diabetes would be to give lie to my life, and to what I stand for. I'm doing what I do in large part simply to show that I *can* do it—despite diabetes—and to inspire others who have the disease.

No, my diabetes is not the reason I'm in a crabby mood. Part of it is pressure. I've got those six other riders competing on my men's team tonight, not to mention my outstanding women's team. I've got our coach here, I've got vehicles and bikes and mechanics, a schedule to adhere to, and sponsors . . . can't forget them. I've got a lot of responsibility, a lot on my shoulders. Plus, I've got to ride, and I'm not feeling really confident tonight because of this injury that has been keeping me up at nights and, worse, keeping me off my bike, so I can't train consistently. I need to get my game face on, and so no, I don't really feel like smiling for a camera.

In the time it takes for these thoughts to race through my mind, however, and before I can even verbalize an objection, my mom's arm is around me, we're grinning for the birdie, and a flash is going off in my face. Darn, she's done it again! Gotten shots of me, and even managed to have a friend of hers get a shot of the two of us in what seems like a nanosecond! A peck on the cheek, a quick hug, and she has moved back into the crowd, presumably to find the best spot to take still more pictures once the race starts.

That's my mom, and as cranky as I can get with her, I have to laugh. She gets it done.

Meanwhile, the frenzy is mounting. More yelling over the microphone about the awesome field assembled for this, the thirtieth edition of the Criterium. In the crowd I notice our new Team Type 1 pro cycling director and coach, Vassili Davidenko. He catches my eye, smiles, and gives me a thumbs-up. I smile back, in part to acknowledge him, but also simply because I am genuinely happy that we've got him on our side. Hiring Vassili (pronounced Va-*silly*) was a real coup.

In bike racing, the pro cycling director is a sort of performance coach. He's not the coach who prescribes the daily workouts designed to improve a rider's fitness, but the guy who really helps them put their fitness into action. He talks strategy, he talks tactics. Vassili is ideally qualified for the job: a 1996 Olympic cyclist, a rider who has competed in the Giro d'Italia—the three-week-long meat grinder that is second only to the Tour de France in terms of prestige on the racing circuit—and now a sought-after coach, he has the capability to bring our pro team to a new level—one closer to him. A native of the Republic of Georgia, Vassili is now a proud American citizen, with a great accent—*"Pheel,"* he calls me—and a vast amount of knowledge and savvy on how to race bikes. That wisdom was in demand; many pro teams wanted Vassili working with their riders, but we were the ones who were able to coax him over.

"What you are doing here, Pheel, is unique," he told me when he decided to accept my offer to become our coach. "First time in hee-story of cycling."

Vassili is rock-solid Russian reliable. Just two hours earlier, before we drove down into the craziness of downtown Athens on "Crit Night," he had gathered the team in his hotel room at the Howard Johnson's off the interstate a few miles away for a brief strategy session on how we were going to approach tonight's race. We all sat together—a bunch of skinny guys in their twenties, with our PDAs, BlackBerries, and iPods for once turned off—to listen to a man who had won this race twice tell us how to attack the Twilight. "This is prestigious race . . . is also very difficult race," Vassili said. He went on to explain the notoriously treacherous Twilight course, which includes a hill on the far side, along Hancock Avenue, a wide-open third turn (watch out for the pothole there), and a downhill right after the last turn, on Thomas Street. If you're first coming down that hill and around that corner—the fourth turn—on the final, eightieth lap, the momentum you get almost guarantees you will win the race, because the finish line is just two hundred to three hundred yards from the turn.

To get into position for that to happen, though, we were going to have to ride smart—and ride hard. "Remember," Vassili said before we climbed into the team van to take us to the start, "I want full gas from beginning."

Now I straddled my Orbea in the VIP area, thinking about Vassili's words and looking around at my teammates. On this day we were a coast-to-coast operation: half our team was racing in California, the other half—I, Joe Eldridge, Jesse Anthony, Ken Hanson, Dan Holt, Aldo Ino Illesic, and Tim Hargrave—was here for the Twilight. I nodded and smiled at Joe, my best friend, the guy who helped build this team with me—and, oh yes, a type 1 diabetic as well. Our friendship developed here in Athens, where we've raced many times, and now that we are back here again, I realize with a twinge of sadness that we are going in different directions. Joe has become one of our key riders; I've become . . . well, what? A guy who can barely can carry his weight, because of a bum leg? I don't want to be riding just because I'm the guy who runs the team; I don't want any favors.

Tonight, I'm racing to survive—something I'm familiar with. In addition to the constant battle of monitoring and regulating my blood sugar, eating and drinking and monitoring and injecting the right things at the right times, I've got to worry about the same damn leg that has hampered me on my bike for the past two years. The problem is in the iliac artery—one of the main pipelines for getting blood into the leg. Due to the stress of repetitive motion in the cycling position combined with all this blood trying to get down through to help feed the working muscles, the artery is subjected to extreme stress. As one doc explained it to me, it can get kinked, like a malfunctioning hose. That's what happened to me. The condition is called iliac endofibrosis; I've had one surgery already in an attempt to fix the problem, and hours of rehab, but it hasn't worked. Now I'm back to square one with it. When I start riding, sufficient blood can't get through the artery, so my left leg begins to go numb, I lose power, and soon I'm trying to pedal a two-wheel vehicle with one leg

How do you give it "full gas"—the 100 percent effort Vassili expects—with 50 percent of your legs?

We're about to find out.

"Put some C-4 on this thing, we're ready to blow it wide open!" cries Chad Andrews, the hyperkinetic Twilight announcer. I shake my head in admiration. I thought *I* was cranked up! How much Red Bull did *he* drink? But I love it. Maybe if more bike races in America struck the right balance between show biz and sport, like the Twilight, we'd have more Americans showing up at our races.

The call-up begins. A dozen of the top riders are introduced. I know most of them. They're neither the revered household names (Lance Armstrong) nor the reviled household names (Floyd Landis) of bicycling, but they're all national-class pro riders. There's Yosvany Falcon, Frank Travieso, John Murphy, Nick Reistand, Mark Hekman. They're representing some of the biggest U.S. teams, as well: Rock Racing, Colavita, Jelly Belly, Hincapie-Barkley (a team co-owned by Lance's long-time Tour de France teammate, George Hincapie).

One by one, they push off ahead of me, out of the VIP area, past the cops holding open the gate, and into the brilliantly lit starting line on the street. It's a blur of colors and logos and lights and cheers. Soon, I'm next on the runway.

"Here . . . he . . . is," says Chad, building up each word as if introducing the combatants in Tyson–Holyfield II. "The founder of Team Type 1 . . . a type 1 diabetic himself . . . and a *baaaaad* dude . . . *Phil Southerland!*"

I keep my helmet off as I coast out to the starting line and wave to the cheering crowd. I want them to see my face, because I want these people to see that Chad is right. I am that rare bird, a diabetic who's a professional athlete. But hey, check this out: I'm that rare professional athlete who also *runs* the team he plays on. I am proud to say that there are few examples in any professional sport of someone who has to take charge of the operation and then take the field, too; a guy who can run the show—and still run the race. But that's what I've been doing since Team Type 1 was a pipe dream right here, in Athens, when I was a college student pedaling around these same streets, in order to get to class on time. We're doing it for a mission—to show what diabetics can do. That's what makes us unique. That's what attracted Vassili and many of the other professionals we've managed to recruit for our team. They get it—this is both sport and something bigger than sport.

"Tonight we got some action!" cries Nelson Vails, the 1984 Olympic silver medalist who's now standing at the start line, next to Chad and serving as a race commentator. With his tailored gray suit and powerful physique, Vails could have easily been mistaken for an NFL running back who's come back to visit his old alma mater. In actuality, he was a short-distance cycling sprinter, one of the best of his era, and you could still make out the outlines of his powerful quadriceps and torso beneath the expensive tailoring.

"Everyone's jacked up!" Vails says. He's right—and now I'm thinking, *Let's go! Enough of the build-up, enough of the hype. We got a race to ride. Let's go, let's go!* The mike is passed to Chad, to finally start the race.

"Get readyyyy tooo . . ." Chad's next words (race? rumble? explode? drink more Red Bull?) are drowned out by the lead motorcycles' roaring into life. I look around at my guys, a quick nod of good luck, and then suddenly the pack is surging, uncoiling. We're off!

The Twilight Criterium is eighty laps; that's eighty times around the center of Athens. You feel like you're in a box, with a tight turn on every corner, and that's part of the mystique of this event. "There are easier ways to make a living than bombing into a tight, pothole-strewn street corner in the dark and hoping to come out the other side upright," observed Joe Silva in *Flagpole* magazine.

He's right, there's a lot of pain, and yet there's also a strange beauty in bicycle racing. In some ways, the pack of riders—the "peloton"—is like a microscopic organism that is constantly changing shape, amoebalike. One lap we're a moving rectangle; the next there's a breakaway attempt, which appears as a long tentacle of riders projecting from a moving sphere. The lap after that we morph into a sort of half-moon shape, as the breakaway is covered and riders and teams vie for position. Ultimately, it's a small triangle being pursued by a large square. The triangle is composed of the three riders in the final breakaway—the guys who gave it "full gas" all the way. The square is the rest of us, our legs screaming for oxygen, our faces grimacing in pain as we watch these other guys pull away. Within these clearly delineated shapes, we are a riot of colors—the various sponsors' uniforms, logos, and bikes making us look like a Jackson Pollock painting with handlebars as we circle the course. This is why cycling is such a cool sport to watch.

Those watching us in the Twilight—and the sidewalks are packed the entire length of the course—are going crazy. Each lap,

I hear Chad yelling on his mike. One time he's screaming, "Preem, preem, preem . . ." Meaning "race premium." Meaning that a little incentive bonus—five hundred dollars—is in play for the first finisher of the next lap. While I would enjoy an extra few hundred bucks, I know it won't be me tonight, so I pay little attention.

Zoom, screech, zoom, screech: that's the pattern as we blast the straightaways and hold on for dear life on the tight turns. I catch a fleeting glimpse of Vassili scanning the peloton, or "reading the race," as he explains it. He's talking on the radio, into our earphones. "Pheel, try to move up." I'm trying. And at first I'm feeling pretty good. But after just five laps, I feel it again, as I have in previous races this season and on all too many training rides: the sensation that somebody has placed his hands around my left leg in a death grip, or tied a tourniquet around my quad, strangling the supply of blood. The flow has been choked to a trickle. I'm now like a cart with one bad wheel: wobbly, uncertain. But I keep pushing, pushing, pushing, gritting my teeth, trying to ignore the pain of effort from my right leg and the numbness in my left.

The signs were there, and they told me I was done. By that I mean literally the *signs*. Posted along the side of the course, by the start/finish line, were a series of billboards promoting the race sponsors, a mix of local and national businesses.

Swagger.us; Velo News; AKO; Jittery Joe's Coffee; WNEG.

I pass them in a blur each lap:

Swagger.usVeloNewsAKOJitteryJoe'sCoffeeWNEG.

And then, after about a dozen laps, as my leg is starting to go numb, they seem to come by slower, slower.

Swagger.us . . . Velo News . . . AKO . . . Jittery Joe's Coffee . . . WNEG.

Finally, with my left leg feeling like a hollowed-out tree trunk,

I have the odd sensation that the signs are going in the opposite direction.

WNEG ... Jittery Joe's Coffee ... AKO ... Velo News ... Swagger.us.

Holy smokes! I'm going backward. Of course, I wasn't *really* pedaling in reverse. It was just that more and more riders were passing me, first making me feel and look as if I were standing still, now losing me, one by one, so that I am now making a steady descent to the end of the peloton. *Is this blood sugar or insulin related?* I think for one panicked moment. No. My glucose-monitoring device is plugged into my arm, and it would've started beeping. Besides, I'd taken my shots, drunk my carbohydrate drink, monitored my blood sugar. No, dammit—this wasn't the diabetes, this was a stupid, if perplexing, overuse injury, caused, so I'm told, by the countless hours spent in the aerodynamic cycling position; the countless repetitive flexes by the muscles of the hips, groin, and legs as they stroke the pedals. Damn that iliac endofibrosis. Has nothing to with my being type 1; although, as an overuse injury, it might have something to with my being a type A, a guy who can't train *enough*.

I could feel myself losing ground, spinning my wheels with one good leg. Finally, I make the decision—the difficult decision that no athlete wants to arrive at. I pull off the course and into the steadying hands of a course marshal, who guides me through a back route to where our team vehicles are parked, a few blocks from the city center. After all that build-up, my race is over in a few minutes.

Depressed and downhearted, I change out of my Team Type 1 racing singlet and bike shorts, slip on a T-shirt and a pair of jeans, and walk back to the finish area. The Criterium and the party that envelopes it goes rolling along, without Phil Southerland in the pack—and despite the frantic manhunt going on in the city's out-skirts while the race is going on. (The body of the professor and alleged murderer, George Zinkhan, was found a week later not far from his abandoned Jeep. He had dug himself a hole . . . his own grave . . . and then fired a shot from a .38-caliber pistol into his head.)

I'm a guy who tries to accentuate the positive, so, after a few dispirited minutes, I try to shrug off what has happened. In a way, I have to: along with my clothes, I now change my identity from pissed-off racer to supportive team founder. Now it's my job to stand alongside the fence and cheer on my four teammates, who are following Vassili's instructions and staying close to the leaders. As the race goes on, it becomes clear that, barring a crash, this will be another solid performance for Type 1, a team that started out as a curiosity, maybe almost as a joke to some people—*"A professional bike racing team of . . . what? Diabetics? Oh, good luck with that"* (smirk). But now we can be counted on to race competitively, and on occasion spectacularly, in every race we enter. On this night, Team Type 1 riders Ken Hanson and Aldo Ilesic finish in fourth and fifth places, respectively—about fifteen seconds behind the overall winner, Heath Blackgrove from San Jose, California, who finished the 80K course in 1 hour 40 minutes and 12.8 seconds.

I applaud them all. I'm proud of my guys; disappointed with myself. Yet, I'm quickly surrounded by well-wishers, old friends, UGA alumni, people from the local racing scene, all congratulat-ing me on the team's performance. Some of them have seen me on TV or the covers of cycling magazines or have read interviews about me in *The New York Times* and *Wall Street Journal*. A couple of people even ask for my autograph, which is pretty wild consider-ing that when I first showed up on these streets ten years ago, as the "snot-nosed" kid cyclist, I was about as welcome by most of the cyclists as a beetle up their bike shorts.

All in all, it's been a good night. I'm delighted by my team's showing. I'm also happy to be back here in Athens, as it runs amok on the greatest bicycling night of the year, anywhere in America, despite the tragic events earlier in the day.

I watch Ken and Aldo get congratulated by the rest of the team, by Vassili, and by our support crew. Soon we'll be spreading the news of our performance here on Twitter, posting it on our Web site and our Facebook page. Our fans, and there are thousands of them, will be sending me congratulations and best wishes and way to go. Way to go? Congratulate Vassili and Ken and Aldo. Congratulate our terrific Type 1 women's team, which finished third overall here; or our guys out West, who had a solid day in their race, as well. But don't congratulate me. I've always been a "reacher"— always reaching or shooting for a level above where a lot of people predicted I should be. I did it as a kid, I did it as an entrepreneur, I've done it as a professional athlete. Part of the key to my ability to make that reach was discipline. I was determined to show people that a diabetic could do any damn thing any other person could do. But right now, I can't. I can't reach the next level as a bike racer and even my discipline and willpower and control over my diabetes can't loosen the iron grip this iliac endofibrosis has on my leg.

A hand is thrust in front of me. I look up—it's a guy I used to ride with years ago. I try to remember if he was a road racer during my college days or somebody I met even earlier, back when I was a kid riding mountain bikes with a bunch of crazy guys in Tallahassee. The bike store we rode out of became as much a home and a school to me as anywhere else; and the mere thought of that store, now long defunct, where I spent so many hours as an adolescent still makes me smile, the way it might have made guys of previous generations or other backgrounds smile over a barbershop, a CYO gym, or the local movie palace.

Yet, I can't quite place this fellow. Did I know him from the bike store? Or at a race somewhere? Or here, when I was a kid tearing up the roads and dreaming big dreams? Regardless, he's one of the guys I've shared that road with, and a friendly face, although the name escapes me. "Hey!" I say, genuinely pleased to see someone from the old days. We exchange pleasantries. He knows about Team Type 1, about our success. He notices I'm in jeans and a T-shirt on a night when I should be in spandex.

"You still racing or are you just in control of things?"

A good question. I take a deep breath before I respond.

"Both . . . sort of."

That word he used—*control*—is something I preach a lot to young diabetics. It may also be the word that defines my existence. My efforts to control my diabetes are nonstop and constant. But of course, the reality is that you have no control when it comes to who you are, where you were born, what you were born with, and to whom. Despite being cursed with a disease that could have killed me, I believe I was lucky in that lottery of life. Lucky to be born in a certain time and a certain place and around certain people.

That's the story I'd like to tell you.

1

A Man from the South

Well it's way, way down where the cane grows tall

Down where they say "Y'all"

—ANDY RAZAF

My name is Phil Southerland. While it's pronounced "Sutherland," the spelling of my surname reveals something about who I really am: a man from the South. I was born in the South, raised in the South, went to college in the South, and still live in the South. You can tell, as a "y'all" or two still manages to creep into my speech.

I've learned from traveling that a lot of people tend to assume that because you are from the South, sound like it, and, in my case, have a name that practically advertises that fact, it stands to reason that you must be a redneck or a right-wing gun nut. I'm none of these. There is not a Confederate flag decal on my bike or a gun rack on my car. I'm not a reactionary or a racist. And I don't get all misty-eyed about the Lost Cause of the Confederacy. Heck, I'm not even that interested in the Civil War, even though I'm pretty sure a few of my ancestors fought in it.

While there are southerners who conform to that stereotype, most of the good people I know from south of the Mason-Dixon line are not like that. I have, however, retained some of what I'd like to think are ennobling and civilized attitudes and conventions of being a southerner. I say "please" and "thank you" a lot and call people I meet "ma'am" or "sir." I do hold doors open for women.

Other southern attitudes have both helped and, maybe, hindered me on my journey. In business, I tend to be a man of my word, and I do believe that there is such a thing as one's "honor" and that it needs to be preserved. On the other hand, I'm pretty stubborn, especially if I think you're forcing me to do something that I don't perceive as right or fair. That's a southern "thing," by the way. I know a few folks down here who would even say that's why we fought that war, but I digress.

My part of the South is a place called Tallahassee, Florida. Yes, Florida. A genuine southern state that has been usurped by snowbirds, Yankees, retirees, tourists, millionaires, and Cuban émigrés. I'm kidding, but really, my Florida has about as much in common with *that* Florida—the Florida of Disney World, South Beach, and Fort Lauderdale—as I do with Gloria Estefan. That part of the state, amazing as it is, in many ways, and as much as I enjoy visiting it, is a long way in every sense from the Florida I'm from. In the Sunshine State, the farther north you go, the more southern you get. In its mind-set as well as miles, Tallahassee is closer to Valdosta, Georgia than to Vero Beach. "Visitors are struck by how southern the city seems," according to one guidebook to what is often called Florida's Great Northwest. "Unlike the more populous parts of the state, Tallahassee is a place where time seems to slow down a bit. People are more easygoing here than in, say, Miami or Tampa. There is an almost genteel sensibility in the air, one that captures the best aspects of southern tradition."

I think they were right on about that. Talk about tradition. Heck, the name Tallahassee itself means "Old Town," and indeed it was already an old Apalachee Indian town by the time Hernando de Soto arrived here in the winter of 1539–40. The Spanish built missions here, and a new tribe of Indians, the feared Creeks, settled here in the 1700s, before their settlements were burned by Andrew Jackson during the Creek Wars of the early 1800s. In 1824, the Old Town was chosen as a compromise site for the capital of the new state of Florida. Why? Because it was midway between the Ochlockonee and Suwannee rivers; and midway between the two established towns of St. Augustine and Pensacola. Tallahassee, located at the narrowest point in that part of Florida, became the compromise—and a somewhat unlikely choice for a state capital, located far from any major river or sea. Yet, that decision affected me and everyone else who would grow up there in the subsequent 185 years—because, although it would maintain its southern gentility and despite its location in the middle of nowhere, Tallahassee became a locus of power, influence, and, most important to me, learning. When it comes to higher education, Tallahassee is to Florida what Boston is to Massachusetts. We have two excellent universities and a community college and, when I was growing up, a quality public and private educational system in which there was one teacher for every twenty students, and nearly 65 percent of high school graduates went on to college or technical school.

So you shouldn't be fooled by the fact that we eat grits and say "sir" and "ma'am" or even by the city's name, which can be rolled off the southern tongue, molasseslike: "Tahhhl-a-hahhh-seee." The truth is that, although the pace may be slow, this was, starting back in the 1980s, a shining example of what people were calling the "New South"; a young city, a smart city, and so, not surprisingly, the place where a smart, young couple named Harold and Joanna Southerland settled down in 1980.

Joanna was like many of those who ended up in the Sun Belt in that period. Her native name was Hagan, and she was no mint-julep-sipping southern belle. Born in Philadelphia, she had moved to St. Petersburg, Florida at age five. Her dad, my maternal grand-father, was a World War II vet—he had served in the navy—and had hoped to make it big in the postwar Florida real estate boom, following in the footsteps of his father-in-law. But he never really did. A kind and gentle man whom I vaguely remember, my grand-father did impart an important lesson to my mom that she passed along to me.

"Whatever you do in life," he told my mom, in one gut-wrenchingly pained and honest moment, "for God sakes make sure it makes you happy."

Clearly, what he had done, with moderate success, had been paid for with the price of a miserable life. My mom initially inter-preted her father's message as "have fun." Which she apparently did at college in the late 1960s. But when she graduated, she ended up finding a job in the most unlikely of places for someone of her independent spirit and liberal views: a steel company. This was pretty funny for a woman who had by her own admission partied her way through four years at the University of South Florida, then traveled for an extended postgraduate European hippie trek, re-turning to the United States with exactly twenty-five cents in her pocket.

But attractive, young, college-educated women were in demand in the business world in those new ERA-conscious 1970s. Joanna worked for a succession of major steel corporations, traveling to Europe and Japan on sales and marketing calls. She would return periodically to Florida to visit her family and friends, including one who had moved to Tallahassee—which my South Florida snob-mom dismissed as "a redneck southern town" (yes, just as those

who were born in northern Florida are proud of its southern lean-
ings, so the folks in South Florida look down when they look
upstate).

In Tallahassee, a young Florida State law-school professor lived
next door to my mom's friend. One day in 1978, he and Joanna
started chatting. "He knew all about Flannery O'Connor and I
was impressed," she recalled. "At the time, I was hanging out with
guys from the steel industry and all they knew about was Budweiser." This guy was also a marathon runner, caught up in the
1970s running boom, which was then reverberating across the na-
tion. Distance runners were cool and sexy and mostly male back
then; and Joanna was impressed. And unlike Joanna, this gentle-
man was from a family whose southern roots were as deep as those
of magnolia trees, as was evidenced by the young man's almost
comically archaic name: Harold Philpott Southerland, Jr.

He couldn't stand "Harold," and of course no one, not even
someone from the Old South, could go around in the late twenti-
eth century with a name like Philpott, so he was called Phil. (Philpott, by the way, wasn't really a first name at all, but rather the
family name of his paternal grandmother.) Phil Southerland, my
dad, grew up in Huntsville, South Carolina. He attended West
Point, did his mandatory service hitch just before Vietnam heated
up, and then attended law school at the University of Wisconsin.
After graduation, he went to work for a conservative Milwaukee
law firm, but he got the boot when he started defending draft
dodgers. Looking back, you have to admire his chutzpah. A West
Point–educated lawyer defending draft dodgers! It revealed an independent, nonconformist streak combined with the time-honored
southern virtue of doing what you felt was the right thing, even
if it wasn't necessarily the best career move. From there Phil went
where really bright mavericks often go: academia. He took a teaching

job at Florida State University's College of Law, which is how he ended up in Tallahassee, charming—with his intelligence, good looks, and reading list—a pretty, young lass sixteen years his junior.

Joanna wasn't the only one impressed by Phil. "He was the kind of professor students loved," she recalled. "Eccentric, brilliant."

And, as it turned out, an alcoholic, whose condition started with a couple of drinks before dinner and got progressively worse. To his credit, my dad would later address his alcohol problem and beat it—as daunting an achievement as anything I would ever face. But in those early years, his manic personality drove Mom crazy. It wasn't only the drinking; as she tells it, he was a man of extremes, often swinging wildly from one end of the spectrum to the other. He stopped marathon running, for example, and instead took up . . . chain-smoking. I guess it didn't help things when I came along. Because what happened then was enough to drive any parent to drink.

I was born on January 15, 1982. From early on in my life, they talked about my baby-blue eyes. They still do. But Joanna saw through that.

Even though I was her first child, Joanna sensed within a few months that there was something wrong: her baby wasn't eating, he was losing weight, and his diapers were always soaked.

Joanna was confident; a bit high-strung and nervous sometimes, concerned about the man she had married, maybe; but sharp-witted and strong. Nonetheless, she was scared. She took me to the pediatrician.

There was something wrong, she insisted.

Nothing wrong, the young pediatrician replied.

"Then why is he losing weight?" she asked, after one week in which I'd lost three pounds.

"Sometimes they do that," he replied.

The situation worsened over the summer. At one point, I started nursing constantly. Joanna called the doctor. "He's probably teething," was the response.

Two nights later, she took me back to him to find out why my breath smelled fruity. He really had no answer.

But over that weekend in August 1982, I began to pant. A horrible sound that made it seem like I was running out of life, already. And for one terrible moment, when Joanna went to attend me, I looked up at her with bright blue eyes—eyes that had only just begun to fix their gaze on the still-new world around them. Those eyes were starting to turn a cold gray—and behind them was an unarticulated but unmistakable cry for help.

She looked into those eyes and saw death. Horrified, she alerted Phil and called the emergency room. "It's probably a flu," said the physician on the other end. "Bring him in."

As they scooped me up, Joanna made one more call: to the pediatrician. "You said it was nothing," she said between sobs. "Well, I'm taking him into the emergency room. You can be there or not."

And with that she wrapped me up and rushed me off to the hospital. There, I was examined. My weight was fourteen pounds, down from twenty-four just a week earlier. I was dehydrated, they said, and put me on a glucose IV—as it turned out later, that was the worst thing that they could possibly have done to me. Within minutes, as Joanna hovered over my bed helplessly, I grew limp and still and began to emit a sickening wheeze. "A death rattle," she recalls today (and believe me, it's scary to hear about this kind of stuff happening to any little baby, but especially when that little baby was you). Panicked, she ran into the hall, calling for help. Orderlies, nurses, and a doctor came rushing in and hovered around the child's bed. "Is he going to die? Can somebody tell me, is he going to die?" cried my mom.

No one could tell her.

They were trying different things. She saw what appeared to be an uncoordinated symphony of hands poking, sticking, and pricking me with various instruments. But again her mother's intuition sensed what they couldn't, almost as if I had sent out a distress signal directly to her. "He was going fast," she recalled. "I could feel it . . . he was dying."

At that point, she was politely but firmly ushered from the room. Never a religious person, Joanna then did what most non-believers do in a life-or-death crisis: she asked for forgiveness and began to pray. They say there are no atheists in foxholes or emergency rooms.

She still remembers it vividly. "It was dusk, and I will never forget the lighting," she told me. "The sun setting behind the steel bars of the pediatric baby bed." It must have appeared as the sun setting on my life. For the next two hours, my father sat in a chair, squeezing the arms until his knuckles where white. Joanna paced so much that the young nurse finally told her she'd be better off if she just tried to sit still. She left, went downstairs, and called her priest.

Joanna was raised a good Catholic girl. Like many of her generation, she had strayed, finding the church too restrictive and in some ways sexist. Now, she wanted to call on the power of the almighty, but at the same time, my mom—bright, rebellious, independent, and now heartbroken—could not rationalize it. Why ask the Lord to save me when he was killing me?

"Why does God do this to a baby?" she cried into the phone.

"Why not a mass murderer . . . someone who deserves it? Or why not me . . . or his dad . . . why an innocent baby?"

He probably gave an answer. But not one that made any sense to her or eased her suffering. As far as she recalls today, "The priest had no answer."

That was the end of her Catholicism.

Two hours passed in a blur. The doctor came in—not the young, self-confident doctor but an old, courtly southern physician. She remembers it was late afternoon when this happened. There were autumn shadows peeking through the half-drawn blinds of the little waiting room. The late-afternoon sky was a pinkish color, an apt metaphor for what she sensed was the darkening of her own life, a life that she was sure would be spent forever lamenting the loss of her firstborn.

The doctor spoke. "I've got good news and bad news," he said.

She braced herself. After what seemed an eternal pause, he continued. "The good news is that he's going to live." Joanna didn't care about the bad news, initially so overjoyed by the surprising report that she began to weep. She barely heard the rest of what he had to say.

". . . But he has diabetes. The youngest case of juvenile diabetes we've ever seen."

Diabetes, she remembers thinking. *Something about sugar and insulin. Injections, right?* No candy bars for her son, she supposed. Regrettable, sure, but he was going to live. Thank God. Then, the other shoe fell. There was more bad news, delivered not that day but a few days later, once a specialist had been called in. He was blunt in his assessment: "The statistics on children with juvenile diabetes this young are grim." Based on then-current care and technology, he predicted that "after twenty-five years, he'll probably be blind and suffer kidney failure—that is, if he's still alive by then."

The dour prospects were based on a scientific truth: high blood glucose levels can end up killing certain cells in the eyes and kidneys, which is why diabetes is the leading cause of adult blindness and of kidney failure. Still this was some prognosis for a young mother to hear about her baby.

Sightless, on dialysis, in all probability dead by twenty-five.

She listened, her jaw set. This time, her reaction wasn't tears. It was quiet, simmering anger, a steely resolve. Her baby boy had survived. And just as surely as she had thought he was about to die that Sunday afternoon in the hospital, she was now equally sure that he would live and continue to live. The maternal instinct that had told her there was something wrong with her child, despite what the first doctor had said, was now channeled into determination to prove this specialist wrong. "Dead by twenty-five, eh?" she said. *Not if I have anything to say about it!* You don't, was the response; there's not much you can do. *Oh yes there is,* she said to herself, driving home that afternoon with her baby. *Oh yes there is. There are days and months and years of things I can do. There are books to be read, opinions to be gathered, lists to be made, friends and neighbors to be mobilized. There* are *things we can do.* Exactly what, she wasn't quite sure at that moment, but she would figure it out. She drove home that afternoon through the rows of cypress trees, past the stately homes and the bustling college campus; back to that "redneck southern town" of Tallahassee, Florida. A town whose merits she would soon be forced to reconsider, for the better.

She looked around at the campus, the hills, the trees, the houses. Her son would live to experience this, she vowed to herself. All of it. Diabetes or no diabetes. I owe her my life for that.

Let me tell you a little bit about the disease that affects me and about 25 million others in the United States alone.

My problem starts with my pancreas, a cone-shaped organ most of us probably couldn't even locate on an anatomy chart. Even more specifically, my troubles began in an area of the pancreas that has one of the most colorful and imaginative names of any part of the human anatomy: the far-flung "islets of Langerhans," which sounds like someplace that Frodo and his friends would have visited in their quest for the Lord of the Rings. Named after the German scientist Paul Langerhans, who discovered them in 1869, it is really a clever appellation for a cluster of about ten thousand cells located in the tail of the pancreas. Amid these cell clusters are beta cells, which function as the microscopic factories that produce insulin—a key hormone in the metabolism of glucose.

Insulin is important because it allows glucose to move from the bloodstream into body's cells to be used for energy. People with type 1 diabetes are their own worst enemies. For reasons that we don't understand, my body's immune system has attacked and destroyed its own insulin-producing beta cells, resulting in dangerously high levels of blood glucose.

This is the "sugar" part of diabetes you've probably heard about. It's interesting how they first figured this out. Centuries ago, they used to take the urine of someone suspected to have the disease and pour it on an anthill. If the ants flocked to it, they knew there was sugar in the urine. In the eighteenth century, the Latin term *mellitus* was added to "diabetes," referring to the sugary taste. But it wasn't until a century later, in 1889, that two German scientists discovered that the pancreas was involved with diabetes. As part of an experiment they removed the pancreas from a dog and found that afterward it urinated again and again. They tested the dog's urine for glucose and discovered that it had developed diabetes— because of the removal of its pancreas.

Something in the pancreas prevented most people from having diabetes. But what? For the next few decades scientists tried to find this magic substance. In the meantime, people tried all kinds of methods to keep diabetics alive. None worked, especially with juvenile diabetics. No doubt, had I been born sixty or seventy years earlier, I most likely would have died, just as the doctor had predicted to my mom. In 1921, a young Canadian doctor named Frederick Banting, fresh out of med school, had an idea. He suspected that cells in the islets of Langerhans played a role; that something in the cells of the islets (or "isles" as they're also called) secreted a substance that was the key to diabetes. He was right—that substance was insulin. Working in the lab of Professor J. R. R. MacLeod at the University of Toronto, Banting was able to isolate it and, with the help of a biochemist, purify and then inject it into a fourteen-year-old boy dying of diabetes. Although already weakened by years of the disease, the young man survived, and with regular injection shots lived for fifteen more years, until he died of pneumonia.

At last, diabetics had hope: something could keep them alive.

In 1923, Banting and MacLeod were awarded the Nobel Prize in Medicine for their discovery of the role of insulin in treating diabetes. (Wanting to give credit where credit was due, the two of them shared the prize with the biochemist, which was a pretty stand-up move, don't you think?)

In the years since, treatment for diabetes has continued to improve. The incidence of the disease, however, has reached epidemic proportions. Here we have to make a distinction: my disease comes in two types. You could call it Diabetes Classic and New Diabetes, and that might be funny, if it weren't for the fact that the rise in the new form has been truly alarming and, unlike my type, largely preventable.

According to the American Diabetes Association, my kind of diabetes—type 1, or juvenile diabetes, which results from the body's failure to produce insulin—accounts for only 5 to 10 percent of the cases diagnosed. The vast majority, and this is where the big increases have come, are type 2—the so-called adult onset diabetes; a form of the disease in which insulin resistance, not deficiency, is the problem. Type 2 is often lifestyle related, with obesity being a big factor.

The ADA estimates that there are now 23.6 million people in the United States with diabetes. That's almost 8 percent of the total population of the country! And it's growing: more than a million new cases are diagnosed each year, most of them type 2. The good news is that the prognosis for children diagnosed with type 1, even at very young ages, has vastly improved in the past decade. A 2006 study in Sweden tracked type 1 children over a period of years and found that not a single child developed end stage renal disease, which is what frequently ended up killing people with type 1 in the past. "That's profound," says Jeff Hitchcock of the organization Children With Diabetes. "It means that our kids will die *with* diabetes, not *of* it." (And when Hitchcock says "our kids," he means it. His daughter Marissa was diagnosed with type 1 at age two and is twenty-three at this writing, and healthy.)

That is a sea change. Meeting the kids that I do at diabetes camps every summer, knowing they can all have a future; a real future, and become whatever they want to be, fills me with joy. It's a far cry from what my mom was facing. Remember, when Joanna was getting the news about me, it was 1982 not 2010 and while things had already changed since the days when a diagnosis of juvenile diabetes was close to a death sentence, there were still no guarantees; and few of the physicians she went to were talking about me having anything resembling a "normal" life. The best that could be expected is that I would survive, not really live. A life of injections and restricted activity; a life limited by a cluster of malfunctioning pancreatic cells.

My mom learned all this in the weeks and months after I was born. Remember, the average age for diagnosis of type 1 diabetes is fourteen. I was seven months old when they figured out that I was diabetic—one of the youngest cases ever diagnosed. Of course, had I been born a few decades earlier, I would have had no chance. But even in the 1980s, when diabetes treatment was already well understood, my odds for living a long and healthy life weren't great. (Losing one's sight is still a concern for diabetics: the ADA estimates that the disease is the cause of twelve thousand to twenty-four thousand cases of blindness each year.)

That was the future Joanna was being asked to accept: your baby boy, quite likely blind and quite possibly dead by twenty-five.

Once she had recovered from the shock, once she was done with the "why me, why my baby?" stage, Joanna got ready to fight back. She knew that diabetes could be managed—meaning that by proper attention to diet and monitoring and taking injections, you could increase the odds of survival and good health. She resolved to do everything she could to manage my diabetes by making my childhood as "normal" as any childhood could be. I wasn't going to get singled out, treated like easily breakable china, or quarantined. Yes, there would have to be changes and modifications in the way we did things. But Joanna wasn't going to let diabetes stop us from being a family or me from being a kid.

Here, what she had originally dismissed as that "redneck southern town" of Tallahassee became important. Our neighborhood, in the Piedmont Park section of the city, was composed of mostly white-collar families, and many of them worked at nearby Florida State University. It was a fairly cohesive place in the early 1980s; not like the Sun Belt suburbs I see today, where so many people are transplants and nobody really knows anyone else. Many of the people we knew had come from somewhere else even then, but we knew them, they knew us, and when news got around that Joanna Southerland's baby was diabetic, they were ready to help.

Believe me, my mom didn't waste any time in taking them up on it.

"Some people are afraid of asking for help," she says. "I'm not."

Joanna drove all over the state, to clinics, symposia, to diabetes-management centers, and made herself an expert on my condition. She went to neighbors and talked to them about the disease. She wanted them to know what was going on if they ever saw an ambulance at our house. And particularly, to those with other small children, she wanted them to know what to do in case I ever had a seizure.

It's interesting how a diagnosis like this affects parents.

My mother got mad, then got motivated, educated, and went on to mobilize the neighborhood.

My father tried to do his best, and as a capable, intelligent man, his best can be pretty good—but not at that point in his life. My diagnosis sent him into a spiral, and he would soon hit rock bottom.

About eighteen months after I was born, my mother took me to the University of South Florida in Tampa, where they had a good pediatric endocrinology unit. Here were physicians who knew kids and knew diabetes.

We spent the day there, as they examined me and did a battery of tests. I think it was a bit of a test for my mom, too—one she intended to ace. She'd already started marshaling her resources to combat this disease. She was staying up nights to monitor my blood sugar. Giving me shots. Organizing my diet and treatment.

She was determined to prove wrong the doctor who had predicted blindness and kidney failure. She was determined to show these guys—the hotshots at USF—that she was a mom who was on the ball and was doing everything humanly possible to ensure that her son was going to live a long, healthy life, despite the early diagnosis of type 1.

She succeeded. At the end of the tests that day, the head physician reviewed the paperwork and looked up at my mom. "He's doing really well," he said. "You couldn't be doing any better than you are now." Joanna beamed as the older doctor shook her hand, then left the room. My mom said she was ready to celebrate, ready to give herself a slap on the back, when she noticed that a second doctor, a younger man, who was doing his residency or internship at the hospital, had remained behind. "He's right," said the younger physician. "Your son's doing fine." He paused. "But you're going to have a nervous breakdown."

As my mom recalls, she immediately crumbled into tears. "I know," she said, through the sobs. "My husband's an alcoholic."

There it was, out in the open, admitted to a stranger no less. My father, the brilliant, charismatic, idealistic, well-read law professor was an out-of-control drunk.

Joanna knew it, but she was so wrapped up in caring for me that she hadn't really faced the issue. But it was clear that father Phil was going down. A few months after I was born, he lost his license and had to take the bus to the university every day. Another time, my mom got a call from her friend and neighbor Iris Yetter. Iris had been driving down our street when she saw me running around the driveway in my diapers, unattended. She stopped, got me safely back into the house, and immediately called my mom. Joanna was furious. I was supposed to have been watched by my dad that day. But he was inside the house, drunk, and I had managed to get out. Good thing I didn't go toddling into the street.

Joanna finally confronted him. She recalls standing in the driveway the morning we left for Tampa, pleading with my dad to stay sober while we were gone—as if he were a frat boy who had a tendency to down a few too many. " 'Please, don't drink,' " she recalls saying to him. "Kind of a ridiculous request, I realize now. But at the time I had no idea how bad his problem was."

We found out later how bad. No sooner had my dad sworn to his wife that he wouldn't drink while she was away, having her diabetic son examined in a hospital, than he walked up to the liquor store with a briefcase, which he proceeded to fill with bottles of vodka. He was lugging this briefcase of booze home when a neighbor spotted him walking, picked him up, and drove him home. The neighbor (who later relayed this to Joanna) noticed the bottles sticking out of his bag. I'm not sure what my dad was thinking— that somehow his lawyer's briefcase would provide immunity for the Stoli bottles peaking out the top? The answer is that in his state, he probably *wasn't* thinking.

At about this time, several hundred miles away, my mom was hearing the words of truth spoken to her by the resident.

According to Joanna, when she started crying, admitting to the young doctor that her husband was an alcoholic, he went on to speak to her directly and in no uncertain terms.

"Then you're just going to have to leave him. You cannot take care of a diabetic and a drunk."

Obviously, no physician today would step over the boundaries of medicine to family counseling, for fear of lawsuits by patients or censure by some medical board. But my mom swears that this is exactly what he said to her. "I'll never forget it," she says of this day.

"I realized that this stranger . . . the young physician . . . was right. I had given up my career. I was totally dependent on this man for finances and for the well-being of myself and our child and he was out of control."

The whole thing with this young doctor seems a mystery to me. She had never seen this man before, and efforts to reach and thank him later were fruitless. No one at the medical center seemed to know who he was. If I didn't know my mom better, if I didn't know that she values truth and honesty and accuracy, I would swear that she imagined the whole thing. But I know she didn't, which is what makes it so strange. It seemed almost as if this physician had been inserted as a plot device in her life, like a playwright deciding that a Greek chorus was needed at this very point to help the audience better grasp a character's motives, or to move the story along.

Which it most certainly did, because instead of driving back to Tallahassee, Joanna decided instead that we were going to my grandparents' house in St. Petersburg. There, she would deliver a long-distance ultimatum to my father. My grandmother—Joanna's mom—was happy to see us. Because she had always been suspicious about my dad's drinking, and sensed that there was more of a problem than anyone was admitting, she fully endorsed what my mom did that night.

Joanna called my dad and said, "I'm not coming home unless you quit drinking."

At this, my dad went off on a real bender. The way I heard it, he got into the shower . . . why the shower I'm not sure . . . and proceeded to drink until he was comatose. My mom, concerned that before long I wouldn't have a father, called a friend who had once been a drinking buddy of my dad's and was now in Alcoholics Anonymous. This fellow was on his way to Europe on business, but he promised my mom that he would get someone over to our house in Tally to help my dad. He did, and they managed to get my dad into a detox center. From there, he went into Alcoholics Anonymous.

So, something positive did come out of this whole awful chapter in our lives. My dad would survive and make a pretty incredible turnaround as he successfully fought his addiction, becoming clean and sober from that point on.

The relationship between my mom and dad was doomed, however, although it would take two more miserable years to finally end.

My dad became immersed in AA. Joanna went to meetings, too, but before long, as she says, "I was Big Book–ed out," referring to the tome that folks in AA read for inspiration and to help keep them from succumbing to temptation. While my mom was home taking care of me, my dad met a woman in his meetings. She, too, was struggling with alcohol, and I guess he felt that she was someone he could connect with better. Before long, as I saw it through young eyes, he started to be around less and less. And when he was, I remember some screaming-bloody-murder arguments between him and my mom.

At some point, probably when I was four or five, Phil Sr. decided to leave Joanna permanently. According to my mom, when he left, he cleaned out all the bank accounts, leaving her with twenty-five dollars. Not even enough to buy insulin for me. One of our wealthier friends heard about it and got so incensed that she told Joanna to go out and hire the nastiest divorce lawyer in Tallahassee, and she would pick up the tab. Joanna did just that. The hotshot lawyer turned out to be a "she"—somewhat unusual in mid-1980s Florida—who immediately filed an emergency motion for support. The lawyer laid out the case, described my illness and how my mom had put aside her own career to devote her full time to raising a diabetic son. The judge awarded Joanna about three-quarters of Dad's salary, so at least she could keep a roof over our heads and insulin in my veins.

One Phil Southerland was now out of the picture. Between diabetes and divorce, the other Phil Southerland was going to have to grow up fast.

2

My Type of Childhood

The team is led by world-class cyclist Phil Southerland, who was diagnosed with Type 1 diabetes at 7 months old. Mr. Southerland has been a trailblazer for people with diabetes and hopes to do for diabetes care and prevention what cyclist Lance Armstrong has done for cancer.

— *THE NEW YORK TIMES*

Long before I ever heard of Lance, I loved *Arthur*.

You know, *Arthur,* the long-running animated kid's show featuring an aardvark with glasses.

I have this vague memory from when I was about six years of age. I'm in my mom's bed, it's afternoon, I'm watching *Arthur* on TV, and then I have this pain in my stomach. Terrible pain. I have to rush to the bathroom. I throw up. I'm lying on the floor by the toilet in a fetal position, crying and holding my stomach. My mom is shoving a glass toward me, saying, "You have to drink something." And I'm saying, "No, I don't wanna."

Then the ominous words: "If you don't eat or drink anything, we're going to have to do the suppository."

That's a threat certain to get your attention, even if you're six years old and can't spell *suppository*. What's being said is, basically, Do this, or we're going to shove a pill up your behind.

The bed-TV-bathroom-puke cycle. This was, according to my mom and my own recollections, pretty much a regular event, from the time I was a toddler until I was about ten or eleven. Every kid gets a cold or flu. But when I got them, things could get serious very quickly. When I got sick from the flu, I vomited. The more I vomited, the less I ate. The less I ate, the lower my blood sugar got. The lower the blood sugar, the greater the danger of hypoglycemia, and my ending up in the ER.

There, I knew, lurked my other great enemy. It wasn't the hospital itself I was afraid of, since I'd probably spent enough time in them already at that point in my life. It was the IV needle. Now, keep in mind that I was no stranger to sharp objects as I had one breaking into my skin four times a day. Diabetics require insulin: my schedule was a shot in the morning, when I woke up; at one in the afternoon, when I came home from school; a third shot at 6:00 P.M.; one more at bedtime.

At first it was unpleasant for me, as it is for most kids. At about age four, I staged an early protest against the inequity of it all, running out of our house and hiding behind a neighbor's house to avoid having a shot. My dad, still in the picture at that point, was unmoved. He came out, found me, dragged me home, and gave me the belt. That was Old South–style child rearing—no doubt the way he and generations of Southerland kids had been brought up. I guess it worked, though, because aside from that one moment of push-back, I took to giving myself injections without too many problems. Here, Dad got credit—it was one of his only contributions to the management of my disease at that point my life, but a very significant one. He had another, more patient side and he showed it when he trained me how to give myself shots. We'd practice using saline. He'd say, "Give me six units." I'd draw up six units. He'd check it. Then I'd dab the alcohol on his skin like he'd shown me, pinch the skin, and inject him. He'd never flinch— even though it must have stung. He was teaching me a skill that I'd need to stay alive, but it was also his way of saying, "See, it's not too bad."

It worked, as I remember a great sense of accomplishment the first time I injected myself. I was probably about five years old at the time. I was in my room, it was time for my shot, and I said, "All right, I'm going to do it the way we practiced it." So I gave myself the injection, and started jumping around the house, "Whoo-hoo! I did my own shot!" My mom was alarmed. "How much insulin did you take?" she asked nervously. I told her not to worry. I knew I'd done it correctly. I also knew that from that point on, I'd be giving myself my shots. It was like the first time riding your bike without training wheels—a big step on the road to independence. Soon, it really didn't seem like a big deal, at all. A small needle, maybe a 12-millimeter-long syringe, pop, and you're done.

That didn't mean I was accepting my disease completely. About a year later, when I was six, I was at a birthday party for one of my little friends, and I asked my mom for cake.

"Sure," she said. "Just do your shot first."

"I don't wanna do my shot. I just want the cake."

"Fine. You'll go blind."

"Huh?"

"Don't do your shot, don't take care of yourself, you'll be blind by age twenty-two."

That got my attention. While to a six-year-old the age of twenty-two seems like a far-off distant time, I was still old enough to be scared by the idea of blindness.

"Okay," I relented. "Can I have my shot, Mom?"

"Nope."

"Why not?"

"Because you're ungrateful. And if you stay that way, you'll be blind by the time you graduate college."

"Okay, I promise! I promise I'll do my shots! I promise I'll take care of myself!"

I don't remember the piece of cake, although I'm sure I enjoyed it. I do remember the impact of my mom's shrewdness. She got my attention, all right. It was a lesson I didn't forget. From about that point on, I took my own shots, and took them faithfully without ever causing a problem. At six years old, I became the CEO of my body.

That IV needle was a different matter altogether. The thing looked like a drill, like one you would see pulverizing concrete during road repairs, except I imagined it boring down into my skin, tearing through tissue and bone, and coming out the other side of my arm. Of course, that never happened, but that's what it looked and felt like in my young mind's eye. The mere sight of that IV needle would always bring tears to my eyes. Mom would say "bite my finger" while they hooked it up. I'd bite so hard, I'd draw blood. So there we were, having blood drawn together. Mine from a giant needle, hers from my little sharp teeth.

One of the little-talked-about side effects of diabetes is the insidious effect it has on the family, how it can erode the bonds among parents and children. Between the parents, it's often the blame game. Because in some cases (although not all) there's a genetic predisposition to the disease, there's a lot of "it's your fault . . . it came from your side of the family!" kind of reaction. Or, if not the genes, it's the way the disease is being managed. Somebody's not doing enough to make sure the child is following the diet; not vigilant enough; not on top of the insulin shots. Blame, blame, blame. Someone's always to blame. As I said, I'm sure the burden of being father to a diabetic child was part of what split my mom and dad apart. But there were plenty of problems there before I even came along. Plus, you pour alcohol on the whole situation, and it's ready to catch fire. Which it did.

By the time I was in elementary school, my father was not around on a day-to-day basis. So the family dynamic was Mom, my brother, Jack, and I. For siblings, the diabetes dynamic can be even worse. The siblings without diabetes see all this attention, all this care being paid to the sibling who has the disease. The kid without begins to wonder: nobody is scurrying around *me,* worrying about every fluctuation in *my* health, every morsel *I* put in my mouth. So in the child's mind it appears as favoritism. That's very typical. To his credit, Jack, four years younger than I, was never jealous—or at least never articulated any jealousy to me or Mom.

He had good reason to get frustrated. There was the time I got the flu—it was another one of those bed-TV-bathroom-puke deals, except it was Christmas Eve. I ended up having to stay overnight and spend Christmas Day in the hospital. My mom wouldn't open gifts on Christmas morning at home because she knew I was lying in a bed in the hospital. So Jack, who was probably four or five years old at the time—peak age for Christmas excitement!—had to wait all day until he could open his gifts; and then he had to do it in the hospital. The kid never complained, and I've always been impressed by that.

Then, there was the time I had a seizure.

Every diabetic lives in fear of seizure—it's what can kill you. These attacks occur when there's not enough sugar in your blood to feed the brain. This typically occurs when you take too much insulin. When I was growing up, there were two types of basal in-sulin (meaning that it's constantly there, working, mimicking your metabolism): One went by the brand name NPH. I used the other one, called Lente. You didn't really have to worry about it. Unless, of course, you were a growing boy or girl and your me-tabolism started to change and your body mass was increasing. Most of that happens when you're sleeping, a time when your blood sugar isn't likely to be monitored. So, suddenly, through no one's fault, the amount of insulin you were giving yourself is inadequate, because your metabolism is changing . . . literally overnight. Remember, insulin essentially takes sugar out of the bloodstream. If the insulin starts taking out too much blood sugar—which it would do when your body was changing—then you'd have a seizure. The first response when that happens is to give the diabetic glucagon, a hormone that causes the liver to re-lease glycogen, which raises blood sugar. To give a glucagon shot, you mix saline into it and then inject it into the patient. So this one time I'm sitting there having a seizure, my mom's calling 911, and little Jack rushes to the refrigerator determined to help. He injects me with saline, forgets to mix in the powder. My mother freaked because without the glucagon, the saline would do nothing, and in a seizure every second counts. So here's a five-year-old trying to help and now he's wondering if he just killed his brother. I can't imagine being in his shoes. Imagine how he felt for that moment: *I might have just killed my brother.* Obviously, he didn't, and the paramedics arrived and gave me glucagon. But what kid should have to go through this?

Jack has had his own problems over the years. In my own way—which is often not very compassionate or gentle, I admit—I've tried to help him. But one thing I sincerely hope is that his ex-periences living in that house, with a diabetic brother and a mother determined to make his life normal, did not inadvertently affect Jack's sense of normalcy. In other words, if he's screwed up (and who of us aren't at one point or another in our lives?), I hope my disease didn't contribute to it. Because he doesn't deserve that. One kid in the family getting his life turned upside down by diabetes is quite enough, don't you think?

At this point you might also be thinking that my childhood was a horror. Puking, injections, seizures, suppositories, divorce, and sibling guilt. A real barrel of laughs. Well, here's the other side of that story. These and a few other episodes stand out in my mind vividly, in part because they were the exceptions, not the rule. While some people find this hard to believe when I tell them, most of my childhood was . . . well, it was *great*. Piedmont Park was a *Wonder Years* type of neighborhood: handsome ranch houses with trees, driveways, patios, and backyards. There, amid the solid suburban middle-class of it all, I did the things most kids of that era did: had fun with my friends, fooled around, played ball, enjoyed video games, watched TV. And although I knew I had this . . . *thing* . . . that the other kids didn't, and I knew I had to take shots every day when they'd get one every couple of years, I wasn't moping around saying "woe is me." In fact, I barely even thought about it.

You see, there's another perspective to type 1. It's not the woe-is-me, this-sucks, I've-been-handed-a-raw-deal perspective, as valid and understandable as that may be. No, in the years since, I've found that I was not the only one who managed to steer a some-what different course; to put the disease in its place, accept what I had to do, and then get on with the business at hand—the business of being a kid. Lots of other young people with type 1 do this, I've learned. Taking this view usually requires a little help and support from others—in my case, the number-one supporter was and still is my mom.

In my case, I know who it is that enabled me to take a bad break and turn it into an asset I could build on: my mom, Joanna.

While it was still the "Morning in America" Reagan years when I was a young boy, my mom was already practicing something that would become a household phrase during the Clinton administration a decade later: that "it takes a village" to raise a child. Joanna had been deeply affected by some of the other mothers of diabetic children she'd met while visiting clinics with me. "These single moms were crying all the time because they had to do it all by themselves," she recalls. "I said, 'I'm not going to let that happen to me.'" She realized that she had to mobilize people around us; she also knew that she would have to take the lead and play the role of recruiter and educator, so that the people responding to her calls knew just what they were expected to do and how to do it.

My mom began doing something a lot of people in her situation are afraid to do: she asked for help. "You'd be amazed how folks will respond when you just ask," she says. "A lot of good people will step up."

A lot of them did. Now, maybe this was good old-fashioned southern neighborliness, or maybe they just felt bad for a young mom saddled with a diabetic son and a husband who had disappeared. But I suspect the same would have been true in neighborhoods all over America. Still, we were particularly fortunate that there were a lot of good-hearted individuals living in Piedmont Park in the mid- and late 1980s, some with kids themselves, others not; some professionals, others blue-collar; some native southerners, others transplants—all of them were ready to help.

The one who still comes to mind first, for both my mom and me, is Sheila Costigan, whom my mom met at the local gym. Joanna—with her limitless energy and type A personality—taught step aerobics at the local health club. Sheila, who had lived in Tallahassee since 1975, took classes with her and became a close friend. Her son Ryan was about my age and was a playmate for me. Sheila remembers the first time Joanna gathered all the moms together for one of her informal "Diabetes Management 101" seminars. "She conducted training sessions, over wine and cheese at my house," said Sheila. "Joanna would talk about glucose, and glucose shock and how to read the symptoms. She'd talk about what Phil could eat and what he couldn't."

I spent a lot of time at the Costigans', who lived just a couple of blocks away. By the time I was five or six, I had learned what I needed and how to test my blood sugar. So I would tell her that I needed a glass of orange juice because my blood sugar level was low. Sheila became sensitive to my needs. I probably didn't notice it at the time, but when she made a batch of chocolate chip cookies, she'd let me take one or two, tell her kids to do the same—and then put the rest away, so I wouldn't feel singled out. When there was cake for somebody's birthday, it was always sugar-free cake—again, done with me in mind. That was a consideration for which I will always be grateful.

Halloween was a perfect example of how my mom and Sheila would collaborate to help make my life seem a little more like every other kid's. With all its candies and sweets, October 31 can be a real minefield for a diabetic kid. You can go trick-or-treating but you can't enjoy the treats, and you feel like an outcast. In order to avoid having me feel that way, Joanna came up with an interesting plan. The neighborhood kids would meet at Sheila's house. Sheila, Joanna, and a couple of other moms would take us all around the neighborhood, as is typically the case in every suburb in America on Halloween. I would go up, dressed as a Ninja Turtle or a ghost or a football player, go door to door, and get my candy along with

Ryan Costigan and all the other kids. But when we'd get back to the Costigans' house and see how much we'd collected—the culmination of every kid's trick-or-treating—Joanna announced that she had a better offer. She'd *buy* the candy from me: twenty-five cents for a piece of chocolate, ten cents for anything else.

Hey, I thought the first time she did this, *not a bad deal.* I knew I couldn't eat that stuff anyway, so why not make some money out of it? I sold my candy to my mom. My friends were watching all this, and the next year they asked Joanna if she'd do the same for them. "Will you buy my candy, too, Mrs. Southerland?" My mom had been hoping they would. Although it probably cost her a little more money than she could afford in those days, these candy transactions were a success on several levels. It kept the sweets away from me, and it kept much of it away from them, as well. After all, while none of them was diabetic, their parents didn't want them consuming all that candy. It ended up making our Halloween a lot of fun, and different from most others. It also become almost like a ritual. The purchase of the candy was made as a group, as if we were the trade ministers of some burgeoning Third World economy dealing with the World Bank. At the end of our trick-or-treating, we'd sit around my or Sheila's house and pool all the candy that we were going to sell. We'd carefully count up how much it was worth and deliver the huge stash to my mom, who would make a big show about checking how much was there. There'd be some haggling, and then finally, after acting as if we kids had driven this really hard bargain, she would sigh and hand over to us what seemed to our eyes a sizable wad of dollars. My friends would squeal with delight over the money, and rightfully so. I remember making between twenty-five and forty dollars, which back in the 1980s was a big stash of cash for an eight-year-old!

My mom jokes today that she may have inadvertently turned a

whole neighborhood of innocent eighties-era kids into the money-hungry hedge fudge managers who helped bring the system down in 2008 through their greed. But it was a good lesson for young-sters embarking on life in a capitalist society, and it certainly helped me feel less singled out because of my disease. It may also have helped to spark my entrepreneurial drive, and the other children learned a lot as well. "Phil taught our kids discipline," Sheila says. "Joanna gave us adults way more than we gave to her."

While that's not necessarily true—my mom and I owe a great deal to Sheila and our neighbors—the discipline Sheila refers to is a steely-eyed seriousness that I began to develop at a young age. While I had plenty of fun being a kid, having the responsibility of being both a diabetic and the "man of the house" forced me to grow up fast. An example of this was food shopping. From early on, Joanna allowed me to watch only PBS. I don't mean *Masterpiece Theater,* but the cartoons and kids' shows like *Arthur* and *Sesame Street*. The reason is that PBS at that time had no advertising at all, and Joanna wanted to protect me from the temptations dangled by the manufacturers of sugared cereals, sweets, and soft drinks. When my brother, Jack, and remote controls came along, that began to change. Soon we were flipping around the rapidly expanding cable dial. Yet, my mom says that when she took us shopping, "Jack wanted everything, Phil wanted nothing." Was it my early expo-sure to advertising-free TV? Maybe. More likely, I had just made the determination that I couldn't eat that stuff, and so I didn't.

If you talk to the people who knew me as a child, they'll tell you that I was "mature beyond my years." I'm not always sure if this is a good thing or a bad thing, but it was undoubtedly a necessary thing. Yes, I was a kid and had fun as a kid, but because of the re-alities of my life—the diabetes and the divorce—I suppose I took on a lot of responsibility early.

Michael Scholl, a friend of my mom's whom she dated for a while, was around the house quite a bit in the late 1980s. He remembers me as this somewhat aloof and quiet kid, with this high-energy mom spinning around me like a dervish, monitoring my blood sugar, making arrangements with the school nurse or the next-door neighbor to help out in this way or that.

My approach was different. I guess I *was* determined: determined to prove anyone wrong who thought I was not capable of doing what any other kid could do, and maybe doing it better. Determined not to let the diabetes rule my life (unless it could help me get things I wanted, like sympathy, favors, and money for my Halloween candy!). Determined to excel, to succeed (although at what, I wasn't sure). Determined to get on with life and to do what had to be done. Above all, though, determined to be a kid—albeit perhaps a slightly more mature one.

I attended Maclay School, a tony K–12 private school about five miles from our house. Located on a one-hundred-acre campus surrounded by a nature preserve, Maclay was founded by a group of parents in 1968. In its mission statement the school declares itself "dedicated to providing a liberal arts education, enabling each student to develop inherent ability to the fullest extent with a balance of discipline and freedom."

My mom liked the sound of this; I think she also liked the fact that the principal of Maclay at the time, Mr. Jablon, lived three doors down from us. His daughter was in my grade, so I got to carpool to school with the principal. The Jablons were part of the solid neighborhood fabric; when my mom got divorced and was struggling financially, they allowed her to continue sending me to the school at considerably less than the regular tuition.

By the time I set foot at Maclay, my mother had thoroughly briefed Mr. Jablon, the school nurse, and all the teachers—probably even the custodian and groundskeepers—about my condition. I'm glad she took the precautions, but fortunately, their readiness was never tested. I recall only one diabetes-related "crisis" at Maclay, if you can call it that. It happened in kindergarten. One morning, my blood sugar was low and I needed to eat in order to bring it back up. So, apparently, I found the lunchbox of my one of my classmates and, while no one was looking, opened it up and ate her lunch. When she discovered her lunchbox empty, the teacher called the class together. "Who ate Amanda's peanut-butter-and-jelly sandwich?" I admitted that I had done it, and explained as best as a kindergartner could that my blood sugar was low. Both my lunchless classmate and my teacher were understanding, which I remember thinking was nice of them.

That's pretty much it. I stayed at Maclay through seventh grade, and what stands out from my years there are . . . well, the same kind of memories you might have. Teachers I liked. Playing football on the playground. My friends. Christmas pageants. Field trips. Nothing really out of the ordinary. But you know what? It's nice to have ordinary memories. It shows that I wasn't standing out in school because of my diabetes. I was just another kid.

At home it was maybe a bit of a different story. I took that idea of being the man of the house seriously. Mom remembers we had this cat named Moon that she particularly loved. But one day a neighborhood dog got loose and caught our cat and killed him. Joanna was mortified; she wept like a baby. I realized that she was in no condition to take care of what had to be done. So, I gathered up Moon's mangled body, buried him in our backyard, and tried to console my mom the best I could. It was hard, and I knew how terrible she felt, but somebody had to be there to do what had to be done.

That someone would be me—then and for the rest of my childhood and adolescence. I guess when you inject yourself four times a day, and regard a trip to the emergency room as a sort of semiannual field trip, other things in life, whether pleasant or not, are put into perspective pretty quickly. Because you had to become sensitive to changes that could happen very quickly in your body—and with life-or-death consequences—you also learned how to size up a bad situation quickly.

There was the time a guy, supposedly a friend of my mom's, came by and put his arm around me in a way that even to me at age nine seemed a little too intimate. I broke free and hid in a neighbor's garage until he left. I don't know what ever happened to him, but I'm sure that Joanna, with her good radar for judging people, made certain he didn't come around anymore.

About a year later, Joanna went out to the West Coast with a guy she was dating. While she was away, she had arranged for my brother and me to stay with my aunt—Mom's sister, Tricia—who was living in St. Petersburg. But when I got there, I sensed that things weren't right. Tricia had her own challenges at the time— she was a single mom trying to raise four kids. The house was kind of a mess. There was no food in the refrigerator. My aunt was going through a difficult period in her life. She was overwhelmed, and I certainly don't blame her for that, but it became apparent pretty quickly to me that this was not a place where we should be. She was simply not able to take care of two more kids, even for just a few days—which my mom hadn't known when she sent us down there. I knew it was best for us to leave. I didn't call Joanna in Oregon, because I realized then there was nothing she could do from there that I couldn't do myself. So I got on my aunt's phone and called Sheila Costigan. Told her the situation, asked if we could stay with her until my mom came back; she said sure. I arranged for a cousin to drive us back to Tallahassee, to the Costigans' house, where we stayed until my mom got home. Although we'd handled the situation, and Jack and I were not the least bit traumatized from spending a day or so in my aunt's messy house, I'm sure I played up the guilt with my mom: "How could you leave us and go out to Oregon with that guy?" In hindsight, I acted like a real jerk with all the guys my mom tried to date. I don't know why I did this, because I needed a father figure. Man oh man did I need one. He would arrive, although in an unexpected way.

3

Fifty Shots a Day

*The man who can drive himself further once the effort
gets painful is the man who will win.*
—ROGER BANNISTER

Through much of my childhood and early adolescence, my mom taught aerobics at the Capitol Racquet Club, near our house. She enjoyed teaching the classes; they kept her in shape and provided her with another outlet for her boundless energy and, no doubt, the frustrations and anxiety she felt being a single parent with a diabetic child.

But while it was good for her, it had the potential to be excruciatingly boring for me. Like I wanted to sit around watching a bunch of what to my eleven-year-old's eye were "old ladies" bouncing around to Milli Vanilli. Luckily, I had an out. Instead of being confined to the child-care area with my kid brother, Jack, I got a free pass. The owner of the club, Benny Chastain, had a son named B.J., who was in my class at school. B.J. needed some company, too, while his dad was busy with the club operations. Sticking with him, I was allowed a bit of a freer roam around the club.

Capitol was like a lot of health clubs of that period. The future for them—and the industry—was in fitness. The second-floor aerobics studio was where my mom taught; the weight room, with its array of impressive machines and barbells, was off-limits to me. But at the same time, racquetball was hot. It was what a lot of people came to Capitol to do, so the courts were where the action was. I'd peer in from the other side of the high glass walls and watch the club's top guys—and some of the best racquetball players in Tally were at Capitol—slam and volley for hours on end. It all looks pretty eighties in retrospect, but these guys, with their short shorts and plastic goggles, slamming and bamming, making acrobatic saves and impossible returns, just captivated me.

One day after school, when one of the courts was open, B.J. took me out. I knew he had played but I didn't know he was good. He put a racket in my hand and served up a ball. The game was over at that point. B.J. destroyed me. His shots whizzed by me like rockets and left me flailing and fluttering away at air. He'd set me up by shooting to one side, then as I lunged to return it he'd simply hit my return back against the wall on the other side. He didn't move a step, and I'd be panting and flustered in a desperate, futile effort to get the shot.

"You suck," he said as we walked off the court.

I already knew I was a decent athlete, despite my small size. I'd been a star at kickball and lunchtime games at school, and I was a fast enough swimmer to win trophies. But racquetball is a game of power, skill, and endurance. Proficiency is drilled into a player. Unlike, say, running or jumping or even throwing a football, hitting a hard rubber ball that's bouncing off four walls with a racket is something you learn how to do. "There's nothing natural about being a natural," writes coach Ed Turner and national champion Woody Clouse in their book *Winning Racquetball*. "You have to work your way into it. In racquetball work means practice sessions full of drills."

I kind of sensed that, even as a kid. I watched the adult players practicing at Capitol; I knew that even B.J. went out on the court diligently and did his drills. But how? What kind of drills? I was ready to do the work, I just needed a supervisor to show me exactly what kind of work to do. I needed help if I was ever going to compete with B.J. Even more than that, I needed someone to guide me a little as an athlete; to support me, to give me some encouragement, a boost up or, at times, a figurative slap down, as well.

In short, I was a boy and I needed a dad.

While Joanna could show me how to be strong, she really couldn't show me how to hit a curveball. Or a racquetball, which was my immediate concern.

I certainly wasn't alone in this. In 1960, 90 percent of American children under the age of eighteen lived with their fathers and mothers. By 1993, when I was twelve years old, that number had declined to 70 percent. This was around the time that the impact of fathers on their children was actually the subject of national debate. The year before, 1992, an episode of the popular TV comedy *Murphy Brown* had sparked a huge controversy when the show's eponymous heroine decided to have a child outside marriage, prompting the vice president, Dan Quayle, to criticize the show for "mocking the importance of fathers." The same day as the show aired—September 21, 1992—an article in the *Washington Post* quoted a researcher from Ohio State University as saying that a child's cognitive development had nothing to do with whether the child's father was present in the household.

This "father flap" led to something good—a spotlight on single mothers, like mine, who were trying hard to raise their kids, often in difficult circumstances. When Diane English, the producer of *Murphy Brown,* accepted an Emmy for the show that year, she thanked "all the single parents out there who, either by choice or necessity, are raising their kids alone."

Those single parents deserved that shout-out. But, as David Blankenhorn wrote in his book *Fatherless America,* the idea that children "don't need" fathers just doesn't hold water. Of course they need their dads. In the book, which was written in 1993, around the time of this national father debate, Blankenhorn alleges that the words of the Ohio State researcher who was quoted in the *Post* article were taken out of context; that his research, in which he analyzed the impact of fatherlessness across race and income ranges, found that those who were harmed most, in terms of behavioral issues and so forth, were Caucasian children, especially boys.

An interesting finding, although I certainly don't need a family-values guy or a sociologist or anyone else to tell me today that it would have been better for me to have had a fully functioning, nonalcoholic father in my life. But I had one dynamo of a mother and a neighborhood-full of good and generous friends. I did well at school and I matured quickly. Where I felt the need for a dad was in my young athletic life. I had been embarrassed by another boy and now wanted to raise my level of play to the point where I could compete with him and possibly avenge that loss.

The man who would shape my life at that critical moment and for the next couple of years was not related to me by blood or marriage, nor was he dating my mom. Psychologists have a name for this kind of adult male who pops up to play a specific role in the life of a fatherless child: the "Nearby Guy."

Some, such as Blankenhorn, are skeptical of the value that this kind of part-time, substitute dad can have. Here's what he says about him: "As a cultural model, the Nearby Guy is a father who is better than nothing. He is not a biological father. He has never been married to the mother. Unless he is a live-in boyfriend, he does not live with the child. He is much more detached and peripheral, closer to being an acquaintance than a relative."

Others disagree. "Many men today were greatly influenced by father figures who were not biological relatives," writes psychologist Jerrold Lee Shapiro in *The Measure of a Man*. "Often these unsung heroes provide crucial male nurturance to youngsters at critical times. Teachers, coaches, big brothers, mentors—all may render the missing ingredients."

That was my Nearby Guy: Kevin Davis. The right man at the right time. No one ever said to me that he was supposed to be my father and I knew he wasn't. But from the first day that I met him—a six-foot-tall, two-hundred-pound guy standing on the other side of the glass of the racquetball court, watching intently as I practiced—I sensed that this older guy was willing to help me and, just as important, knew *how* to help me.

Kevin was married to Holly, who, like my mom, was an aerobics teacher at the club. Also like my mom, he was not a native of Tallahassee. Although you would never guess it to hear his drawl now, Kevin was born in Rockland County, New York, but had moved to Florida as a kid. There, he was raised by a single mother—more of a rarity in his day than in mine—and yet excelled at sports. He moved to Tally, he jokes, "to chase a girlfriend." He ended up going to Florida State University and after graduation got a job teaching at a high school just outside of Tally. He started doing real estate on the side and within a couple of years had earned his license and become one of the most successful real estate brokers in the city.

Kevin and Holly had two young sons at the time I met them. He may have sensed that my mom needed help and felt bad for her; or maybe he wanted to practice being a dad, as he waited for his older son, a toddler then, to grow up a bit. I do know that what-ever the motivation, it came from the heart, and Kevin has a big heart. He took pity on the pint-size kid trying to hit balls against a wall and falling on his face. Modest guy that he is, if you ask him today about the role he played in my life back then, he'll play it down: "Hey, here was this cute little kid with all this drive and motivation. He didn't seem to quit and he clearly wanted to get better. So I tried to help him a little bit."

It was a lot more than a little bit. Kevin became my Nearby Guy, my surrogate sports dad and then some. "Kevin was a god-send," my mom says. As far as I was concerned, he was the com-plete package: big and strong, but gentle; confident and competent, but kind and generous. Once he took me under his wing, I felt protected in a way I hadn't before. I also felt that if I did exactly what he said, I'd be as successful as he was. And he *was* successful: I have vivid memories of him walking around the club lobby, a racket in one hand and one of those boxy, early-nineties cell phones in the other, talking to clients, cutting deals, and making the mys-terious world of adults seem intriguing. As far as I was concerned, though, Kevin's most important credential was his prowess on the courts: he was the best racquetball player in the club, everyone knew it, and now he seemed willing to share with me some of his secrets.

The main secret was simple: work.

"Racquetball is a sport of angles and repetition," wrote Woody Clouse. "Practicing drills is the only way to obtain the consistency needed at the highest levels. The amount of time you spend work-ing on your racquetball skills will dictate your degree of success."

Kevin knew that, as well. He understood that achieving profi-ciency in racquetball, as in so many other things in life, is simple: you have to practice. Practice the shots, practice the return, learn the angles, understand the geometry of the game. The first day he offered to work with me, Kevin took me onto one of the courts and, with shocking ease, began hammering the ball against the wall and returning it as he talked. I was bug-eyed as I watched him shoot. "How do you do that?" I asked. Kevin smiled. "By doing the same things I'm telling you to do."

The goal for me was to hit fifty shots a day for each type of common racquetball shot—short, long, forehand, backhand, cross-court, and back and forth. Fifty shots a day; and with each one, I'd try to get them to go lower and lower to the ground. Kevin was teaching me to perfect the "home run swing" of racquetball—the kill shot, the unreturnable shot, which guaranteed points for him who could master it.

I was determined to become a great killer.

Almost every day over the course of that winter, I practiced dutifully the way Kevin had asked me to. After school, I'd come home, do my homework, take my insulin shot, and then drive with my mom to the club. She'd go teach a class; I'd make a beeline for the courts. Kevin was usually there and would spend a few minutes with me, check my progress, offer me tips. Then I'd spend about two hours practicing; the sound of the rubbery *thunk* of the ball hitting the wall and then bouncing off the floor back to my racket was my accompaniment. When about twenty minutes of this had passed and I got bored, and began thinking it might be a lot more fun to be watching TV than hitting shot after shot, I imagined B.J. sprawled out on the court after his vain attempt to return my game-winning shot . . . the shot I was honing right now. I imagined Kevin smiling and nodding in approval.

That kept me going. I was only about eleven years old and a long way from physical maturity, but I was beginning to develop a mental toughness that would serve me well later.

After a few weeks of the drills, Kevin announced that I was

ready to start practice play. There was a challenge court for A- and B-level players at the club. Kevin was always on the A-court, beating all comers; he set me up on the B-court. I felt like Robin to his Batman, although in the comic book of my life, Robin was getting the stuffing kicked out of him—at least at first. The B-level didn't correspond to age, just ability. So my competition was often adults, and even without a lot of racquetball skills, their superior reach, size, and strength allowed them to dispatch me easily. For a while, at least. As the weeks and months rolled by, the practice and the play began to coalesce. The proficiency I was developing from *thunk-thunk-thunk*ing the ball fifty times a day in practice began to pay off. I started scoring points against my opponents and sometimes beating them.

Kevin would smile and pat me on the back as he marked this progress. He wasn't a big rah-rah guy; but he didn't withhold praise, like some men do, in the false belief that their silence will somehow make them appear stronger. I was a kid, I was working hard, and part of the reason I was working hard was to please Kevin, my sports dad. So a "good job" or a "way to go, Phil" from him meant a lot more than it did from anyone else.

There's a mind game in racquetball that I began to appreciate. The trick in that sport—like most volleying games—is always to keep the other player guessing. You have to anticipate where your opponent is going and you have to expect that he thinks he knows where you're going to go, so you've got to be thinking two steps ahead. Kevin helped me here. We developed a series of signs, much like a catcher with a pitcher in baseball. If he held up an index finger, that was a backhand. Two fingers meant a lob serve. A hand slash meant a kill or a cross-serve. So, as the play started, I'd look out at Kevin, standing outside the B-court, looking in through the glass, and get the sign. More and more, they started to work.

As much as I wanted to please Kevin, I also wanted to cream my friend B.J. Understand that this is the mind of the eleven-year-old boy at work: I considered him a pal, and we'd hang out sometimes. But he'd embarrassed me on the court (and rubbed it in a few times, since); plus I sensed that he'd been handed a lot of things in his life on a silver platter. He had money, a father, security, and new equipment and new clothes whenever he wanted them. I was motivated, I suppose, by pride and jealousy, but boy, was I motivated.

Kevin knew that beating B.J. was my goal. He also knew that B.J. was a good young player, so he encouraged me to play against him from time to time. At first, I wasn't sure—I didn't want him wiping the court with me again. But, after a few weeks of practice, I mustered up the courage to get out on the court with him. He whipped me, 15–1. I didn't cry, didn't throw my racket on the court, but I was frustrated. I seem to remember worrying that, after my shellacking, Kevin would take the racket out of my hand and break it in two, or suggest that maybe I should look for a new sport, because clearly I was hopeless. Nothing of the sort. "Don't worry about it," Kevin said after he heard I'd been stomped by B.J. "Just keep working, keep practicing. It's going to pay off eventually."

His confidence in me, his positive attitude, kept me going. A couple more weeks went by—eight different drills, fifty shots per drill. Serves, backhands, forehands—you name it, day after day. At this point I was begging my mom to go to the gym even on days when she wasn't teaching aerobics. Soon it was time for another game with B.J. I took another trouncing, but this time I managed to string together a couple of longer volleys. I noticed him panting at one point and sensed that I had made him work a little harder for his victory. More practice, more days of eight drills, fifty shots per drill. Another game. This time it was 15–4, and I got a few good shots off against him. Then 15–5. I sensed that B.J. was probably starting to think twice about playing me now, but he had his pride, and he was a confident athlete, with good reason. He was the best kid on the racquetball court in one of the biggest racquetball clubs in the city. And the next two or three times we played, he managed to keep me at bay. Again, 15–5, 15–6.

"You're getting close," Kevin said, as he encouraged me to keep up the practice. He also started talking tactics with me a little more. Things like the crosscourt shot, where if you and your opponent are on one side of the court, you try to hit the ball near the center of the front wall so that it will angle all the way across the court to the far back corner—impossible to return. He taught me more about when to try a kill shot (when you are in forecourt or center court and your opponent is deep) and when not to (if the ball is above the knees and you try to kill it, it could rebound high off the floor, giving your opponent time to get to it). This was a lot for an eleven-year-old brain to take in: shots, angles, timing, anticipating your opponent's moves—while you're moving at top speed. But I began to get it; I began to move my game up from the basics to a more competitive level. (Looking back, I also realize it was strangely similar to the "diabetes game.")

One afternoon, several months after I'd first picked up a racquet, B.J. and I squared off on court B. It was late afternoon, after school, and there was no one else around, so I didn't have an audience. Too bad. We played one hard-fought game. I don't remember too many of the particulars except that it came right down to the wire and I hit a corner kill—a shot Kevin had taught me and that I'd been practicing for weeks—and beat him 15–14. I remember jumping for joy, and B.J. angrily storming off the court. And I remember the big smile on Kevin's face when I told him. "Way to go, Phil," he said, putting his hand on my shoulder. "You worked hard, and you did it."

I could tell that he was really happy, really proud of me.

My relationship with Kevin Davis extended beyond the racquetball court: he took me to a couple of football games. He knew I was a big Florida fan—a heretical stance to take in the city where the Florida State 'Noles (Seminoles) inspire an almost religious devotion among the community, and longtime coach Bobby Bowden was regarded as a sort of secular saint. I think Kevin recognized my contrary Gator allegiance for what it was—a little independent streak—and took me to a Florida game in Gainesville. This was an exciting introduction for me to big-time sports. He also took me (and a couple of other kids, including my arch rival, B.J.) boating on Lake Jackson. And come springtime, he volunteered to coach my Little League, so I had my "dad" as my coach there, as well. He was a great teacher there, just as he was on the court. Our team made it to the playoffs that year and several years hence, and I know that every one of my teammates was a better player and a better person for having been under Kevin's wing.

After beating B.J. at the club, I began to play racquetball in citywide tournaments and even traveled to compete in a couple of state championships. Kevin drove me to some of these—my mom, still my number-one fan, came as well—and I remember it was at one of these tourneys that Kevin had to abandon his role as my quiet, behind-the-scenes supporter and come out vocally on my behalf, which was not his style.

In one of these round-robin tournaments, I was paired up against a guy in his late twenties. He walked onto the court, saw me, and asked angrily, "What are you doing here?"

I said, "I'm here to play."

"I'm not playing you . . . you're a kid."

He stalked off the court and started making a scene.

"I didn't come here to play this kid. Look at him . . . he's like two feet tall."

At that point, Kevin interceded. "Hey," he said. "Why don't you just play the kid? He might surprise you."

"Come on," the guy said.

"No, you come on," Kevin said, gathering his full frame up in an imposing stance, as he stared this guy right in the eyes. "Instead of running your mouth about this kid, go out and let your racket do the talking. I know him, and I can tell you . . . he's not going to cry if you beat him. And that's *if*."

"All right," said the guy, as he shrank back from Kevin.

We played, and while I'd love to tell you that I whipped a guy in his twenties when I was pushing twelve, that's not what happened. He won. But it was close—I suspect a heck of a lot closer than he thought it would be. I remember that at the end of the match, he couldn't get off the court fast enough. Kevin winked at me.

"Nice game, Phil."

I said thank you to Kevin Davis that day and I'm still saying it today.

4

Revolutionary Spirits

We get them all at RAAM, intellects, nuclear scientists,
housewives, tuna fish salesmen and whack jobs.
—RAAM BLOG 2007

One of the many lessons I learned from Kevin and racquetball is that hard work produces results; that the more effort you put in, the more success you achieve. I was still too young to realize that that formula isn't always perfect or fair, but at that point in my life, when I was still a shy kid, self-conscious about my small stature and probably about my diabetes as well, it helped guide me to my real calling as an athlete.

But first, it helped me take better charge of my diabetes. During one of my regular visits, my endocrinologists told me my A1c was 8.1. It was the first time I had heard of the A1c, or at least the first time it registered with me. "Does that mean I'll go blind?" I asked, echoing the fear I'd harbored since I was six.

The doctor couldn't look me in the eye and say no, so he tried to be as honest as he could to a kid. "With this number, I can't promise you that you won't."

I let that sink in. "So where does it need to be?" I asked.

"A little lower. Maybe seven."

"Fine. What do I need to do to get it there?"

He reiterated the basics: don't eat food when your blood sugar is high; take your shots every day; and so forth.

It was mostly what I had been doing, and while I don't believe he recommended exercise specifically, I was starting to become more active in racquetball and other sports, as well. When I came back three months later, it was a little lower: 7.4.

"Will I go blind from this?" I asked again.

"No guarantees. But you're doing better."

I knew what it was like to go from being bad to better—to success. I knew from Kevin Davis what it took to climb that ladder. More work, more vigilance. Three months later, I went back to the doc. My A1c was down to 6.8.

I remember him reading the result, then smiling as he looked me in the eye.

"You're going to see."

That was it. From then on, my A1c checks during my every-three-month visits to the endocrinologist became my Diabetes Report Card. A lot of people with type 1, particularly then, didn't even know what an A1c was. I'd made it my goal—like being able to toss a football fifty yards, or bash a ball over the centerfield wall, or run a mile in under five minutes. Keeping a low A1c became almost a motivating force for me, and it would inform my diabetes management from then on—even as my interest in sports began to change.

Although I would continue to participate in team sports, including a brief stint in football where I served as an undersized tackling dummy for a bunch of oversized young rednecks, my success in racquetball, my drive and eagerness to work hard at it, was moving me toward the sport that would define my life.

People often ask me when I started riding. Truth is, I can barely remember a time when I *wasn't* riding something. It's like that for most American boys and many girls growing up in the suburbs. We're pedaling around on vehicles from the time we're toddlers: Big Wheels around the driveway, tricycles on the sidewalk in front of the house, then kid-size bikes with training wheels up and down the block. I do have a distinct memory of my dad helping me make that transition to a two-wheeler. He did it in his own inimitable way, and looking back I hope he was sober at the time, although his method did work, regardless. I was probably about five years old, and I remember him guiding me along with his hand on my back, our first time without training wheels, and we came to a hill. The hand, instead of providing support, became a prod, giving me a sharp push. "Okay," he said, as the bike started to roll downhill, "now *ride!*" I made it 300 yards, and crashed, but picked myself up. And did it again and again.

I kept riding, all over the neighborhood, throughout my childhood. But around the summer of 1994, when I was twelve, the rides began to get a little longer. Then I got a great Christmas gift: a Roadmaster mountain bike. My mom had bought it at Walmart for about $150—a lot of money for her in those days. It had eighteen speeds, cool purple and green colors, and although it was a relatively cheap bike, I thought it was the best thing ever. With my mighty Roadmaster I began to boldly venture forth in the neighborhood. I wasn't racing yet, or riding crazy trails with it. I'd make bigger loops, pedal down unfamiliar streets, explore new areas— local parks and trails that I'd never known existed.

Often, I rode with a group of friends who lived in the area. One of them was a very cool guy named Johnny. Johnny knew stuff that most of us kids didn't. One day, he and I rode all the way up to Lake Overstreet in northern Tallahassee. Located in a state park (the former property of Alfred Maclay, the namesake of the adjoining county and my old private school), the area is well known to birders, hikers, and joggers. The 144-acre lake itself is accessible only by trails, which made it even more intriguing. When we finally got to the lake, we were exhausted. We leaned our bikes up against a live oak, plopped down by the water's edge, and enjoyed a breath of lake-cooled air that swept over us. To my astonishment, Johnny whipped out a pack of Marlboros and lit one up. "Want one?" he said through clenched teeth, offering me the pack. "Uh . . . sure," I said. I took it, accepting the match that Johnny had at the ready, inhaled—and felt an intense burning in my throat like I was going to throw up. I wanted to cough, but I held it in so I wouldn't look like a rube.

"First time?" Johnny said.

"N-no," I sputtered, emitting a cloud of smoke. "Well . . . yeah."

Johnny just laughed.

We went back to Lake Overstreet a few more times that spring. Each time, we'd sit on the shore and light up. Soon, I was inhaling, not coughing—and proud of it. One time, Johnny brought fishing poles and showed me how to fish. He knew stuff like that—stuff you needed a dad to teach you, preferably a dad who owned an RV and spent a lot of time in bait-and-tackle stores. When Johnny caught a largemouth bass, he showed me how to clean it and then built a little fire and cooked it up. There was no end to what he could do, and I was mightily impressed. If you believe that our lives are threads that can be spun in various ways depending on the circumstances, I suppose that one scenario for the life of Phil Southerland is that I'd still be sitting on the banks of Lake Overstreet today. There I am, in this alternate life, sipping a Budweiser, waiting for a tug on my line. Maybe Johnny, now potbellied and tattooed, is sitting right next to me, offering me yet another Marlboro. That didn't happen, fortunately for me, because my diabetes would have been out of control in no time with that kind of lifestyle. What occurred instead was that one night, after we got back from our Lake Overstreet smoke-and-ride, his mom found his cigarettes in his room. That was it. Calls were made, voices raised in two households, and punishments administered. I was forbidden to hang out with Johnny. I rarely saw him at all after that and never smoked a cigarette again. To this day, I can't drive by the signs for Lake Overstreet without feeling a burning sensation in my throat.

Still, I kept on riding, with a different crew. The J Gang plus P: Joel, Jacob, Jack, and Phil. I forget how we all met—when you're a kid, there's rarely a specific moment of introduction; you just always seemed to have been around one another, in school, in Little League, or just hanging around the neighborhood. I do remember the first time we rode together. It was a Friday after school in late spring, they all had cheap but sturdy mountain bikes, like me, and we did some long loops around the neighborhood. They were good riders, they didn't get tired or bored after a half hour like some kids, and I liked them. The next week we rode on Friday, and then Saturday. The week after that, we rode the entire weekend. We weren't riding that hard, just pedaling along at what I'd call today a conversational pace. But we weren't looking to converse, we were looking for adventure, something new and exciting to stir up those languid, Tallahassee afternoons.

One day, we found a trail that started behind the local Winn-Dixie supermarket. A new trail was big news for us, so we picked it up right away, and before long we'd come to a creek. I wasn't a fast rider at that point, but I was becoming increasingly bold on the bike. When we came to the creek—which was about four feet wide—the four of us pulled up alongside one another, and looked at one another, as if saying, "Well, who's going to be first?" I didn't hesitate. I wanted to prove myself to these guys, show them that I might be little but I had big balls (I really didn't at that point: puberty was still a few years away). I backed up a few yards to give myself some momentum, and went pedaling as hard as I could and . . . *whoosh* . . . lifted myself and the Roadmaster over the creek, coming down hard on those knobby tires on the other side. "Yeaahhh!" I shouted, fist pumping. The other guys followed. We might as well have just reached the summit of Mount Everest.

Those kinds of peak moments were the exception, however. Usually, we just did our winding loops around Piedmont Park and the adjoining neighborhoods. For hours we rode through the hot Florida summer. People began noticing us. One of them was a guy named Andy Roberts, who was probably in his late twenties then. "It seemed like everywhere you drove that summer, you'd see this group of kids riding their mountain bikes," Andy recalls. "I'd be like, 'Who are these kids? It's a hundred degrees and they're out riding? What are they doing?'"

Later, when I got to know Andy, I told him why we were out there in the blazing heat of the deep South. We were kids, we were bored, school was out, and we were too old (or broke) to go to summer camp and too young to hold summer jobs. So this was what we did. Today, maybe we'd be sitting in an air-conditioned room, playing XBox or having our conversations on Facebook. Back then, we rode mountain bikes in the heat, endlessly. But there was another reason that kept me out there.

I really wanted a Snickers bar. Yeah, I know it sounds silly, but remember, I was thirteen years old, and despite all my mom's best efforts, I was now at the point where I was getting sick and tired of not being able to eat or do what I wanted because of my stupid diabetes. I wasn't so stupid that I thought I could just ignore it or stop taking my shots. I just wanted a damn candy bar like everybody else! The insulin in those days took two hours to work, and I didn't have the patience for that. Instead, I'd jump on my bike and ride until my legs started feeling tired and sore. Then I knew it was time to eat. And by that point, a couple of hours into the ride, I began to realize that I'd probably done enough exercise that I could actually eat that Snickers bar without throwing my blood sugar into a tizzy. It was all instinctive, not very precise or scientific, but it seemed to work. I figured that as long as I was riding a long time and eating when my body told me it was hungry, I'd be all right. Plus, I wouldn't have to hear from my mom, "Did you take your shots? Did you check your blood sugar? Remember you shouldn't eat this, you shouldn't eat that. . . ." Bicycling became an escape from my usual routine; it afforded me a way to be with friends and see cool new places and have fun, and, on top of it all, it allowed me to have a Snickers bar.

The timing of this two-wheeled wanderlust was good. As an adult, I've learned from diabetes educators that at about age thirteen or fourteen, the disease often takes a turn for the worse. Because that's when kids—most kids, whether they have diabetes or not—typically start to rebel. Instead of growing your hair long or blasting loud heavy-metal music in your room, the best way for a type 1 adolescent to rebel is to let your diabetes control go to hell. Guaranteed that if your mom or dad sees a blood sugar of 300 day after day, they're going to flip out—and with good reason. I didn't go that route. I pissed my mom off plenty; not doing the dishes, which was one of my obligatory chores, was one big weapon in my adolescent rebellion, and not doing my homework was another. I suppose also that my vanishing for most of the day, day after day, wasn't doing much for her peace of mind, either.

But my form of rebellion or adolescent expression—bike

riding—ended up helping me to control my diabetes. That wasn't the main reason I was riding my bike, and I certainly didn't do it to please my mom or hold myself up as some model of adolescent type 1 propriety. I just wanted what every thirteen-year-old boy wants: a little more freedom, a little more control over my own life. Bicycling was my way to do it. And I figured out quickly that in order to keep on doing it, I had to stay on top of my disease. If my blood sugar got too low, I'd feel weak and wouldn't be able to ride with my friends as long. If I let it skyrocket, I could go into a coma or my kidneys could shut down. So I kept paying attention to it, not because I was supposed to but because it was a means to an end.

Above all, I loved to ride. And mountain bikes were such a great way to ride. You felt like you could conquer any terrain, anywhere—and for a kid, particularly a diabetic kid whose life is prescribed and restricted, the feeling that a mountain bike gives you, that there are no limits, that you can go anywhere, was intoxicating. Plus, you could do tricks and demonstrate attitude and prove that you were just too cool for school—also very important for adolescents. On top of all this, it was a good time to be a mountain biker, no matter what your age. In the mid-1990s the sport was going through a renaissance. Mountain biking had started in the 1970s in California, when some adrenaline junkies converted their old two-wheeled cruisers and balloon-tire bikes into indestructible downhill-racing machines. That was what the sport was in the beginning: they would throw these jerry-rigged bikes into a truck, drive up to the top of a mountain, take out them out, and then race down. According to a history of the sport on Mountainbike.com, they'd use coaster brakes, which would get so overheated during the descent that they would have to be repacked with grease before the next ride. Crazy stuff.

By the early 1990s, mountain biking had spread nationwide and was no longer a purely downhill endeavor. Up hills, over boulders, across fields of jagged rocks . . . whatever the obstacles, mountain bikers loved them. At the time I started riding, the mountain-biking community was abuzz with the first X Games in 1995, which featured a mountain-bike race, and the upcoming introduction of the sport to the Atlanta Olympics in 1996. Mountain biking had arrived, although I think most of the guys I knew who were riding at the time thought the X Games were way cooler than the Olympics. They cultivated this off-road-rebel attitude that became synonymous with the sport, and as a rebelling adolescent, I figured I'd fit right in.

I was right.

It was in the spring of 1995 that I drove with my mom to Revolutions, a store in Tallahassee that specialized in mountain bikes. Perhaps it was because I was doing a good job with my diabetes. Perhaps it was because she felt guilty about my even having diabetes, an emotion that I, like a lot of type 1 kids, callously exploited. Whatever the motivation, I'd managed to persuade her to get me a new bike. Revolutions was located in a cluster of shops right across the street from a bar called Paradise, off Thomasville Road in a part of town that was, shall we say, off the beaten tourist path. Owned by a guy named Kent Whittington, they had just moved into these digs—a beat-up World War II–era building—a month earlier. There was a good ol' southern shade porch in the front, and as I walked in I noticed a Foosball table in the back. *Foosball?* I thought. *Wow. Working in a bike store must be a great gig.*

There were a lot of guys in the store, but no one seemed to be buying anything. They were sitting around in their bike clothes— they must have just come back from a ride—talking about races and riding and bikes, arguing about what kinds of brakes and tires were superior to others. They ignored me and my mom and continued their banter. The riders called one another by nicknames such as Bigworm and Bike Ape. The whole scene was bizarre but fascinating, almost as if we'd stepped into a strange colony of alien creatures with hard-shell heads and feet with grommets on them.

"Hey, folks, can I help you?" said a cheerful voice. I looked up to see a giant towering over us. Chris Slaton was his name and he would become one of my best friends, even though I doubt he or I would have believed that at the time. He was six feet two inches tall and weighed about 220 pounds. I wasn't even five feet tall yet and weighed barely 100. A long ponytail snaked around his shoulders. He looked like he'd just stepped out of a heavy-metal music video.

"I . . . I . . ." I stuttered.

Joanna stepped in. Six-foot-two or no, mom was never intimidated by anyone and always prepared to take care of business. "Hi," she said. "We'd like a mountain bike for him. He's thirteen, rides a lot, and we want something good, but not too expensive." Chris (who still remembers this day) guided us over to a bike made by Barracuda, a Colorado-based mountain-bike manufacturer that made a strong bike with a smaller frame, which was perfect for me. They also were ahead of the curve in that they donated part of the money made from every bike sold to some charity that was helping to save the rain forests. My liberal, NPR-listening mom liked that and so did I. I took a test drive. The Barracuda seemed custom-made for my diminutive frame; it had a lot of stability and maneuvered well, too.

Mountain bikes then weren't nearly as sophisticated as they are now. Take the tires. Today, a set of really nice tires—and they have tires for every kind of terrain or condition—costs nearly as much as the first bike I raced on. In a way, I'm glad I started when it was a bit simpler. I couldn't have afforded a pair of semislicks with side knobs *and* spiky tires with widely spaced knobs *and* all the other tire combos available to mountain-bike riders today—or, for that matter, the advanced "damping" systems or pedaling platforms they now have that control the speed with which your suspension can compress. Hell, I barely understood what a suspension system even was back then. I just wanted a bike that was comfortable and cool-looking and durable enough to do what I wanted to do. The Barracuda was my ride.

"This is the one for me," I said, as I braked to a halt in front of my mom and Chris, who had been chatting amicably outside the store while I tooled around on my test ride. While I didn't realize it that day, I was buying into something bigger than a new mountain bike. I was about to become part of a group—okay, call it a "subculture"—of adults that would really change my life.

A couple of days later, I rode my new Barracuda back to Revolutions, accompanied by my three J friends. "But we don't have any money to buy anything," protested Joel, when I suggested we head over there.

"I know," I said. "It's just a cool place. Maybe if we're quiet they won't notice us and we can still check it out."

They did notice us, but no one seemed to care that we weren't there to shop. I soon learned that very few of the guys who hung around there had ever bought anything at Revolutions. In fact, a couple of times, when real customers did come in, I heard the guys recommend other bike stores in the vicinity as being far better suited to their needs. The gentle giant Chris was the only guy who seemed to be working. He did everything there: he built bikes, fixed bikes, sold bikes. On weekends, and often after work, he'd have an audience. "I'd be working," Chris recalls, "and nine guys would be sitting around, just hanging out."

As a business model, Revolutions was a flop. But as a place where kindred spirits could gather, exchange information, and enjoy one another's company, it was fantastic. There was a refrigerator in the back and, on weekends, a cooler full of adult beverages. Revolutions was also a bit of a nuthouse, not surprising considering the characters who congregated there, as well as the general characteristics of mountain bikers, who tended to be guys who loved throwing their bikes and bodies around for fun. They were up for anything. The second time I saw Chris, the ponytail was gone and the top of his head bristled with a razor-sharp crew cut. "What happened?" I asked. "Oh, I got overheated during a race," he said. "So we figured the hair had to go. We shaved it off in the back of the store."

Heads were shaved at Revolutions, and balls constantly busted, as well. By the third time my buddies and I showed up at the store, they had started making fun of us. One particularly mouthy guy— another giant of a man—heard my name and started referring to me as "that little Philbert." His name was Ray McNamara, and he was the chief wise guy in a store filled with them. Originally from Texas, Ray had followed a girl to Florida State, but by the time I met him, he had settled into a rather eccentric career as a flea market vendor, selling as he puts it "any kind of junk I could get a good deal on." Although he was in his early thirties when I met him, Ray had, like me, come to mountain bikes recently, and he still likes to joke that "Phil and I are the same bike age."

While I can laugh about stuff like that with him now, back then Ray was kind of scary. Standing well over six feet, he also towered over us, but, unlike Chris, he would order us around, make us run errands, pick up food or sodas for him and his buddies. One time Jacob, Joel, and I were wrestling, just horsing around in the store, and Ray and some of the other guys decided to use it as an opportunity to have some fun. So they made a big show about proper decorum in the store and how we teenagers were scaring away customers (there were no customers, but that was beside the point). Ray came up with a creative punishment. He duck-taped a square on the floor, barely big enough for the three of us to stand in. "Now stay in that box and shut up, or we're kicking you out of the store," he barked. I'm sure he and Chris and the other guys could barely contain themselves from laughing as three of us—Joel, Jacob, and I—stood there contritely, as if we were in detention. I'm also sure they thought it would last just a few minutes before the three antsy adolescents would beg to be let out. What they failed to take into account was my determination, how important this all was to me. By now I had realized that Revolutions—and by extension this world of long, adventurous mountain-bike rides and the giants who rode them, the freedom it represented to me, and the excitement and joy I derived from it—was where I wanted to live. Nothing was going to keep me away, certainly not a square of duck tape. So I hunkered down like a contestant on one of those challenges on the TV show *Survivor,* where they make everybody stand on a greased pole for hours on end. The last one standing wins immunity. Well, I won immunity that day. Joel and Jacob couldn't handle it, they begged for early release from the box, and as punishment were sent off on some kind of ridiculous errand for Ray or made to clean out the old, dirty bathroom in the back of the store. But I stood there with my arms folded, stone-faced, as the minutes ticked off. Took all the fun out of it for Ray and his coconspirators, but I think I might have earned a little respect that day at Revolutions.

Crowded as it was with bicycles, parts, and big riders sitting around, you couldn't really bike *into* the store—although it was known to happen during some of their drunken parties. The three-foot-high porch in front of Revolutions, however, intrigued me. Mountain biking is partially riding, partially jumping, and partially (this might be the biggest part) having the nerve to try crazy stuff. Stuff like doing a three-foot-high vertical jump with a bike attached to you. That became a goal: on late afternoons after school, I'd ride over to the store and try it. I remember trying, trying, trying. Then trying some more. Couldn't do it. After a few weeks, I figured out the trick. First, I'd lift up the front wheel onto the ledge. Once the wheel was up, it was all about popping the back of the bike upward and forward at the same time. Doing this in one motion required squeezing every muscle in my body, firing every muscle fiber that an adolescent body could muster in one massive, muscle-contorting, bone-rattling explosion.

Figuring out the trick to the jump wasn't the same as mastering it. Sometimes I'd get one wheel up but not the other and I'd have to hop off the bike or land on my keister, which I did a number of times. Luckily for me, I had a short memory, particularly at that time in my life, because when that happened I'd just bounce back up and continue trying. I kept trying and trying, practicing and practicing, just like I'd done with racquetball. (*Fifty shots a day*, I could hear Kevin Davis telling me, in my mind.) The night I finally nailed that jump onto the ledge happened to coincide with a party at Revolutions. It was a Saturday, and because I was still too young to drink beer like everybody else, I drifted out to the porch to continue my quest. Once again, I began trying to make the jump, going through the now-familiar motions that were becoming almost second nature. Front wheel up (lift!), back wheel up and forward (pop! squeeze!), and suddenly . . . I'd done it! I jumped three feet and landed my bike . . . *slam* . . . front wheel down . . . *bam* . . . the rest of the bike up and over the ledge, the old floorboards creaking and whining.

"Yes!" I said triumphantly, raising both arms over my head.

"You're a persistent little bugger aren't you?" I looked up and saw Ray leaning against the doorframe, grinning. "I've been watching you. Not bad, Philbert, not bad. Now go get me a Coke." Ray recalls that night, as well. "I saw him out there on the porch, and thought to myself, *Ha, look at the kid trying to do this,*" he says. "I started watching him. He kept trying and trying and trying, and I remember thinking that he was determined to do it, and damned if he didn't. And that's what it was like with him. You couldn't get rid of him. He was like the bike-shop pet. Every time I went into Revolutions, that little Philbert was always there."

Although Ray could be an ornery cuss, he had a good side to him, as well. He was smart and had a wit as razor sharp as Chris's new crew cut. He was also generous with his time and money and advice, and, like the other guys I began to meet in the store, he became part of this zany, extended family that had adopted me. It was as if I had suddenly discovered a house full of big . . . really big . . . brothers and uncles. They were the Revolutions crew and gradually I became part of them. So what if I was more like a mascot, as Ray liked to call me.

The crew did more than just hang around and make fun of one another, however. They rode and they raced, and some of them, I soon learned, were among the best mountain bikers in the Southeast. The weather in Tallahassee is conducive to riding—it never gets too cold there, and while we don't have mountains, we have plenty of rolling hills and miles of trails I was starting to explore. The Revolutions guys had a regular Sunday ride, thirty to forty miles through various parts of the extensive trail network that surrounds the city. The first time I was asked along (after much pestering on my part, I might add), I was almost too excited to speak. I—the kid, the pet, the mascot—was being given the opportunity to join the giant mountain-biking men of Revolutions on their weekly ride! Now I was going to show them that I deserved this honor.

That part didn't work out so well at first. On the Sunday rides there was a B-group and an A-group. The B-group was comprised of guys who liked to ride for fun. The A-guys were the serious riders and included most of the core group from the store. I figured for sure I'd be able to hang on to the B-group. What I didn't reckon on was becoming a one-man C-group. Within just a few miles of leaving the shop that Sunday, I found myself falling behind everybody. Before long, I was all alone, just my bike and I. At that point, I realized that we were on a trail that cut through a park near my house. The thought entered my head: *I could just turn off here and head home.* It would have been a big decision. I could only imagine the abuse Ray would heap on the little Philbert who had cracked on his first Revolutions ride. I'd be standing in a duct-tape box for weeks. I might never have even worked up the nerve to go back to the store again.

Maybe, I thought for a moment as my spirit and body began to flag, maybe this wasn't for me. Maybe I had gotten ahead of myself here and should just go back to doing loops of Piedmont Park with guys my age. I was just seconds away from turning the handlebars of my Barracuda off the trail and toward my house—and what could have likely been a new direction in my life—when I saw a familiar figure heading back down the trail.

"How you doin', buddy?" It was Chris, the gentle giant, with a big smile. "Come on, ride with me."

I forced a smile in return. "I'm good, I'm good," I said, unconvincingly. He knew I was lying and that every word I spoke would cost me energy that I needed to keep going, so he just chatted away as we pedaled along. I learned about Chris's life, how he'd started out as a skateboarder before bicycling. He told me how he'd first seen a mountain bike around 1990 and wondered "what the hell is that?" but how he'd then become enamored with the big knobby tires and wild colors, and was now a hard-core mountain biker. Because I was still at an age when I thought that all adults had always been doing whatever job they were currently doing, I was shocked to find out he'd actually been something before becoming a bike mechanic at Revolutions. Chris was a gifted photographer and wanted to make that his life's work. He'd even gone to school for it, before he realized that had he become a professional, he would have lost the joy and the freedom of shooting whatever pictures he wanted, whenever he wanted. So now he was in graduate school for business, while working at the store.

I listened to him talk as I pedaled along with all my might. We hit a steep hill, and I wasn't sure I could get up. But about halfway through the climb, I felt myself moving faster. I turned and saw that Chris had leaned over from his bike and put his hand on my back. He was pushing me up the hill. "No problem, buddy," he said, smiling. "That's what friends are for."

Chris truly was a friend. Of course, that didn't mean he was above making fun of me, either. That was the basis of everybody's relationship in the Revolutions group, and being the youngest and smallest, I was the target for a lot of it. On that first ride, when we finally caught up with the rest of the group, who'd stopped for a quick water break, I was showered with abuse.

"Hey, the little kid is here."

"Are you sure that's not a midget on that bike?"

"What's the matter, Philbert? You got diaper rash?"

And that was just the stuff I can relate without making this an R-rated book. Soon enough, though, I got to the point where I could give it as good as I could take it. I learned how to make fun of guys' mothers, their riding abilities, their personal hygiene. Juvenile as it sounds—and it was undeniably juvenile—that was the way the Revolutions rides were: a sort of high school locker room on knobby tires. But I loved it, even the insults. I like to think I was always personable as kid, but I was still pretty shy. These guys, with their banter and their teasing, helped me come out of shell and made me more confident. On those Revolutions rides, I improved as a cyclist, but more important, I grew as a person, as well.

I became a regular on those rides and looked forward to Sunday mornings, even though for most of that year I was usually one of the last finishers. But that didn't break my spirit like it almost had on that first ride. Instead, I used it as fuel to help me get stronger, better. My riding began to have greater purpose—instead of looping around the neighborhood, I was now training to do better on the Sunday ride, and to prove myself to the Revolutionaries. Ride by ride, slowly but surely, I began to pick it up. I measured the improvement in small increments and would set little benchmarks for myself every weekend.

The first week, I'd been dropped after about twenty-five minutes of riding. So I set my goal for the second Sunday: *This week I will hang with the pack for thirty minutes.*

And I managed to.

The following Sunday: *I will stay with the pack for forty-five minutes.*

And I did.

The Sunday after that: *I will attack, and get to the front of the pack at least once during the ride.*

And I attacked and got to the front.

Having those little milestones was crucial and kept me going. Best of all, my progress was getting noticed. Soon I was ahead of most of the B-group and hot on the trail of the studs. The A-group guys must have sensed the determined kid who was working hard to catch up with them, Sunday after Sunday, because they started regrouping at a couple of points during the ride, waiting for me to catch up before continuing. One Sunday, Dave Desrosiers, one of the really fast guys, came over to me during one of those designated "Southerland Stops."

"You know," he said, "it's a pain in the ass waiting for you, but you're fighting so damn hard, we don't mind. If you weren't trying, we wouldn't wait."

Another A-team rider was appreciating my progress, as well—the same guy who'd first noticed me pedaling around the neighborhood with my buddies the summer before, in the hundred-degree heat. Andy Roberts had a sort of "dual citizenship" in the Tallahassee cycling world. You'd see him at Revolutions from time to time, and he'd often join us on the Sunday ride. But he was also a road rider and hung out at the rival bike shop in town—a shop that went by the rather uninspired name of Joe's and catered more to the roadies. Being a mountain and road biker in those days was like being a driver in both NASCAR and Formula One racing. They're both automobiles, they both race around a track, and the similarity ends there. Same here: mountain and road bikes are different, mountain and road races are different, and mountain and road riders are very different. (Think Lance Armstrong in his yellow jersey pedaling down the Champs-Elysées, and then picture some guy no one ever heard of, covered in mud in the middle of the woods. See the difference?) Andy was that rare cyclist who managed to thrive in both worlds (and as I would soon follow in his footsteps, I took careful notice of how he did things). He had started riding mountain bikes because he'd read that it would make him stronger on the roads. He kept coming back because he enjoyed the Revolutions guys, the camaraderie, and the whole laid-back, rebel atmosphere of mountain-bike racing, which was different than you might find in the traditional and more more tightly wound road-racing world.

Andy had an aunt who had diabetes so he was a little more sensitive and attentive to that, as well (even though, as I tried to do in every aspect of my life, I didn't want anyone making a big deal about it, especially not the Revolutions guys). Later, Andy would admit that when he realized I was type 1, "I got a little worried. I didn't really know about would happen to Phil on a three-hour ride. Would he drop off the ride, would he collapse and go into a coma? I wasn't really sure how a body reacts to that kind of effort."

To be honest, neither did I. My long neighborhood rides had taught me enough to know that I wasn't going to keel over—and that I *would* get to enjoy my Snickers bar!—but on the Sunday rides with Revolutions I was pushing it to a new level of intensity. I'm proud to say that after riding with me a couple of times, Andy sized me up this way: "Phil was total determination." I was focused on getting better, and Andy was willing and able to help. He was a really good teacher. One of his many insightful tips was the admonition to "scrape the gum off the bottom of your shoe." The first time he said that, I looked down at the cleats of my bike shoes, thinking that maybe I'd stepped in a wad of Wrigley's spearmint on the sidewalk. But no, he was speaking about the circular motion you use with your feet that, while biking, allows you to use your hamstrings and glutes as you pedal, recruiting more muscle fibers and helping you become 2 percent more efficient. That may not sound like much of an improvement, but consider this: over a three-hour ride, a decent mountain biker will probably total about 16,000 pedal strokes. If your muscles are working 2 percent more efficiently, that's 320 fewer strokes over the course of a ride—a lot less energy expended.

Some of our Sunday rides would take us into the Munson Hills, south of town. The 7.5-mile trail, laid out on an old railroad right-of-way, wound through the Apalachicola National Forest. Like a lot of our rides, it was beautiful: we'd ride traffic-free through lush woods full of pine, cherry, sassafras. Looking back, I confess that I probably wasn't as attentive to the natural riches around me as I should have been. I was too focused on the bike and the banter. But if you were on a mountain bike the Munson Hills *forced* you to pay attention, because the so-called hills are actually large sand dunes—remnants of a shoreline formed there aeons ago. The terrain was fine, sugary sand, and if you held on too tight and rode it the wrong way, you'd sink into it. Andy told me the trick was to ride light on your hands and feet so that you would "float" over the sand.

Soon I was floating across the Munson Hills.

The Sunday rides stoked my competitive fires. But I knew that those rides were designed to get the Revolutionaries in shape for the races, particularly in spring and fall. This was where they took all their hard-won fitness, their finesse and their balls-to-the-walls attitude, and put it to the test. I wanted to test myself, too, and prove myself in front of my new family. So I pestered them to take me along on a race, and finally, in the spring of 1996, they agreed. A group of them was going to compete in the Thunder Mountain Classic in Thomaston, Georgia, about three hours from Tallahassee. Did I want to come? Boy, did I. I raced home on my bike and begged my mom for permission. Please, please, please, let me go. Joanna realized how important this was becoming to me, and once she heard that Chris Slaton, whom she trusted, would be there, she gave her approval—along with a lengthy list of dos and don'ts involving my care.

She might not have granted permission had she known the kind of conditions we'd be traveling and living in. Bike racing in those days and at that level was about doing as much as possible for as little as possible. None of these guys was rich—they were, after all, still in their twenties, for the most part—and so any way they could save a buck, they would. On the Friday afternoon before the race, about twelve of us piled into someone's SUV (bikes strapped on top or on the back or wherever else we could fit them), and breaking just about every vehicle safety and occupancy law in two states, we drove up to Georgia. Everybody was there: Chris, Ray, Dave Desrosiers, most of the Sunday-ride crew, and a few girl-friends and wives as well. When we arrived, we pitched tents on a campground about four hundred meters from where the race would start the next morning. Later, after having fueled up on a cheap dinner of fast food, we sat around a campfire, the guys drink-ing beers and telling dirty jokes. I sat with a bottle of water and thought how great it was to be a fourteen-year-old mountain-bike rider with the guys from Revolutions.

It's funny: while I remember that night, and the trip, very well, I can barely recall the race. I know the course was seven miles and featured a couple of tough hills, including one climb that was a mile and half long, but not much more. I was in the juniors divi-sion, which meant I was competing mostly against guys sixteen to eighteen years of age. They were all bigger than I (who wasn't?) and stronger, and while I think I rode respectably, what was more important to me was that I didn't embarrass myself. I didn't—and what I remember vividly was the great postrace atmosphere: all of us riding back in the car, Ray cracking us up with funny stories about what had happened to him during the race, everyone's high and low points. They're the bike racer's versions of war stories, and to hear them and be part of them for the first time was a wonderful feeling, a camaraderie that I had never felt before. If this was bike racing, I wanted more of it.

TWELVE HOURS OF THE ROCK

By the time I turned fifteen, in January 1997, I'd done a season of mountain-bike racing with the Revolutions guys. I'd probably been in about a dozen races in Florida and Georgia and had moved up in the rankings from beginner to sport (the third and highest level was expert). I'd won a juniors race, beating the kids my age and earning the respect of the older guys. While Ray still called me the Revolutions mascot, even he seemed to acknowledge that I was now one of them. I loved racing and the idea of going longer and longer began to appeal to me. So when I heard that a promoter was organizing a twelve-hour endurance event in central Florida, my ears perked up. This was big news! No one had ever heard of a twelve-hour mountain-bike ride before. Revolutions was abuzz with this, and when Jeff Sukach, one of the riders, invited me to be part of a three-person team in the twelve-hour competition, I eagerly accepted. However, it turned out to be a quick trip. On the very first lap of the race, held in what was called the Hard Rock Cycle Park—actually a converted limestone mine—Jeff crashed and broke his scapula. We had to drop out and I was really upset. I had been psyched for this race and was developing a single-mindedness, maybe even self-centeredness, about my cycling. I was finding it too easy to overlook someone else's misfortune—in this case, Jeff's. If you hindered my efforts, got in my way of achieving a goal, look out. Not a particularly admirable trait, but one that I'm told is common with driven people, especially young ones trying to prove something to the world, as I most certainly was.

The day after our aborted race efforts in Ocala, I was in the shop, running my mouth about how we'd made this trip for nothing, about how I hated being dependent on other riders, I'd have been better off just doing it myself. Kenny Williams, a solidly built African-American rider, challenged me.

"Hey, Phil," he said, "if it's such a problem for you to be on a team, why don't you ride that twelve-hour race yourself next year?"

"Okay," I said, "I will."

"No, you won't. A twelve-hour solo ride? What are you, fifteen years old? You can't do that."

Somewhere in my mind, bells started ringing, sirens screamed, klaxons roared. I hated being told that I couldn't do something. Couldn't eat candy, couldn't beat B.J. in racquetball, couldn't live past twenty-five.

Kenny was a nice guy. He was a police officer in Tallahassee, so he carried the weight of authority with him. He didn't come around that often to Revolutions, but when he did, I remember he was always friendly, always made me laugh. But not at this moment. He'd challenged me. I looked at him through narrowed eyes and spoke through clenched teeth.

"I can do it."

He grinned back at me. "I got a hundred bucks says you can't."

"What?"

"You heard me. I'll bet you a hundred dollars that you won't do this race."

I may have gulped. Considering that I was still living on an allowance of about ten bucks a week, there was no way I could rustle up a hundred bucks on a lost wager. But that didn't matter, because I didn't intend to lose or pay him anything. I was going to do something that no one in Revolutions, and few people anywhere else in the state of Florida, had done. I was going to ride twelve hours straight on a mountain bike.

"You're on!" I said, and we shook hands.

By this time, 1997, biking was the most important thing in my life. At age fifteen, kids start going to parties, hanging out on weekends. Not me. I spent Friday and Saturday nights at home because I had early bike rides the next morning. On the weekends, most self-respecting teenagers were asleep until eleven or noon. By that time, I'd already been on my bike for three or four hours.

I'm sure it was weird to a lot of my classmates at Ponce de Leon High School. Bikes? That was kid's stuff. If you wanted to be a man in Tallahassee, you got a car. And I was almost at the age where I could do that. Except for the fact that there was no way we could afford a car. So I kept riding the bike. By this time, I had added road biking to my repertoire, and that was about to open a whole new world to me. But the twelve-hour mountain-bike ride in Ocala, the hundred-dollar bet, was still my major focus.

I think I know why Kenny Williams was ready to make that bet. I was still a little bantamweight, still looked like a twelve-year-old boy even though I was now a fifteen-year-old teenager. Heck, I was the last guy to go through puberty at Leon High. Kenny knew I was a single-minded little cuss . . . by then, everybody at Revolutions did . . . but he probably still figured that if I didn't have hair under my armpits yet, there was no way I was strong or tough enough to ride half a day on a mountain bike. Maybe he thought he'd teach me a lesson about being so cocky.

All that kept me going; all that was in the back of my mind as I went through a second season of mountain-bike racing, and some road racing, too. The event—the 12 Hours of the Rock race—was scheduled for February 1998, and as the date approached, I began to realize that not only was this race going to be a decisive moment for me as a bicyclist, it was probably the culmination, the swan song of my life as a mountain biker. I was becoming increasingly attracted to road cycling by then. I began to realize that this was where the real action was, where the best cyclists and biggest races were. I was starting now to think less about the Munson Hills and more about Alpe d'Huez in the Tour de France.

But whether I was riding a short, squat mountain bike or a sleek, lightweight road bike, I knew the twelve-hour ride was going to be the ultimate test for me, the hardest thing I had ever done on a bike. I knew that I had to be ready. After Christmas, I really started to crank up the training. Three weeks before the race, I turned sixteen years old and logged twenty hours on the bike. The week after that, I put in twenty-four hours, which included two six-hour rides. As soon as I got home from school, I'd hop right on the bike and ride until it was dark and then keep riding some more, down dimly lit streets. Oftentimes I was alone on these rides, and as the shadows fell over Tallahassee, I would think about respect. *I'm going to prove 'em wrong,* I said to myself as I ground out the miles. *They said I couldn't do this, and I'm going to prove 'em wrong.* The hundred bucks were almost beside the point, although I certainly wanted to collect. What was much larger than the C-note was the chip on my shoulder.

At the end of that twenty-four-hour week, I felt really strong on the bike. After one last six-hour ride on the Sunday before the twelve-hour event, I decided I was ready. I didn't pick up my bike for the week leading up to the race. Instead, I behaved like a normal teenager: I'd come home and plop down in front of the TV. In hindsight, it might not have been the best training method; but for

a just-turned-sixteen-year-old who'd never done that kind of training before, and was putting his bike and his body through things
that no one—certainly no diabetic—had ever done, resting was
probably the right thing to do.

It worked, as I woke up Friday feeling fresh and ready to go.
I'm not sure how I got through school that day—at that point, it
seemed unimportant compared to my bicycling. But at 3:00 P.M.,
Jeff Asbell, one of the Revolutions guys, pulled up in front of my
mom's house. Jeff had volunteered to drive me down to Ocala and
serve as my "feeder," or helper, during the race. Jeff was a bit of a
rarity among the Revolutions crowd: he was a good ol' boy, and
proud of it. But, unlike most rednecks, he loved to ride his bike. Jeff
was also another of the many good souls at Revolutions. I don't
think he'd grown up with a dad, either, so I think he wanted to be
there for me. Also, like everybody else at the store, he'd heard about
the bet, and I think he just wanted to see how it would work out.

We drove down to Ocala, Jeff and his girlfriend in the front
seat, giggling and blasting the radio, while I hunkered down in the
back, all serious as usual, thinking about the race. When we got
down there, the first thing I did was take my bike out of the back
of Jeff's van—by then, I was riding a spiffy Kona mountain
bike—and go for a spin around the course.

The Hard Rock Cycle Park is about two hundred acres of
densely wooded land located on the site of an old limestone mine.
Years of mining had removed the sand, leaving a clay surface that
was ideal for mountain biking. But since the mine had been abandoned back in the 1950s, nature had reclaimed the ravaged ground,
so it had the look and feel of a forest. "If you parachuted in," says
race director David Berger, "you'd swear you're in North Carolina,
except with a few palm trees." On top of that, the excavations of
the mine operations had left the terrain scored and hilly, with steep

hills and sharp declines as well as sharp turns and many single-track areas.

The next morning, we lined up for 12 Hours of the Rock. Teams and individuals would start together at 10:00 A.M. and ride until 10:00 P.M. At the start, Berger reminded us that you could begin your last lap as late as 9:57 P.M. and it would count as long as you finished the lap. I just prayed that I was still on the course at 9:57.

Today, twelve- and twenty-four-hour races are fairly common, but in early 1998 this was a bold new concept. Twelve Hours of the Rock was the first twelve-hour race in Florida and one of the first in the Southeast. Only a few were brave or crazy enough to try to ride a mountain bike that long over terrain that hard—and none of them was sixteen years old. If you're going to ride a race like this, you have to have a sense of humor. Yet, when I look back today at the entry list for the race, my dead-seriousness leaps off the page. Competitors in 12 Hours of the Rock were given the opportunity to provide a team or nickname on the entry list. Most riders were happy to do so, declaring themselves, next to their real names, as Mountain Chicken, Dog Tired, or even Carolyn's Solo Rock-on Adventure.

What did I put down under the space for team name or nick-name? "Southerland." Creative, right? Yet, totally indicative of my dead-on-serious state of mind that weekend.

The gun went off and we all ran a quarter mile to the start, where our bikes were lined up. While I had trained hard, I really had no idea how to ride this race. For once, even my mentors at Revolutions couldn't help me, because none of them had ever done a twelve-hour ride, either. The best Ray, Andy, Dave, or Chris could offer was . . . *don't go out too fast.* Made sense to me. So as riders went blasting past me, I just stayed in a comfortable cadence, a moderate-intensity pace. No need to rush, after all, because I was going to be out here a long, long time.

I finished the first lap, second, third lap. Jeff and his girlfriend were at the checkpoint each time. "All raht, Phee-yul," he said. "Lookin' gooood!"

I nodded back. I was feeling good, too.

My mood changed a few more laps into the race. We were really in unknown territory here when it came to my diabetes (who knew how it would respond to twelve hours of hard riding?), so I decided to pull into the "pit"—an oversized tent where riders could stop to eat, drink, or tend to their bikes—and check my blood sugar. It was a disturbingly high 400—and when I asked Jeff for my insulin, he realized he'd left it back in the car. I threw a minor fit, as he bolted out of the tent and back to the parking area to retrieve it. As he did so, I tried to calm myself. *Don't panic,* I thought. *Don't eat anything now, just drink some water, and you can get your insulin after the next lap.* So I hopped back on the bike and started pedaling. I was still angry at Jeff for having not had my insulin when I needed it, but I ended up riding my fastest lap of the day.

If I was doing that race today, and I took a shot of insulin, my blood sugar would have dropped down within the time it took me to ride another lap. But with the slower-acting insulin I had back then, it took two, maybe two and a half laps—about twelve to fifteen miles of riding—to really have an effect. But that was the last time I checked my blood sugar. Instead, I got into my rhythm and just kept on going, ticking off lap after lap. I drank water bottle after water bottle. I ate peanut butter and jelly, and Hammer gel, which was new back then.

The course was really muddy, and when it's muddy, bike parts wear out quickly. Brakes go. Sprockets go. And, I noticed, as dusk began to fall, people were starting to go. Soon, I noticed, there were fewer competitors. And many of those still out on the course were starting to look spent, haggard, slouching on their seats, or taking an extra-long time at their aid stations. Meanwhile, to my surprise, I was feeling stronger and stronger. People began noticing that. I started to hear some words of encouragement from spectators in the pit or standing in the dark, off to the side of the trail.

"Hey, kid, nice going,"

"All right, junior, you go for it."

"Stay with it, son, stay with it."

Around six o'clock it started to get dark. I'd finished ten laps—sixty-six miles, or nearly the equivalent of three of our Sunday Revolutions rides back to back to back. Incredibly, we were in the home stretch. I picked up the pace just a bit, to see what I had left, and it felt okay. I started passing some of the solo riders ahead of me. One by one, I was advancing up to the head of the pack, although I really couldn't sense exactly where I was, until the final lap. At that point, Jeff and others on the course started shouting out to me, "You're in second place!" There was one guy, I knew, who was way ahead of all of us. His name was Massimo Cavalli, and as soon as I heard it, I said, "Forget it." Some Italian pro stud, no doubt, who was visiting or had relatives here in Florida; no way I was going to catch him. Besides, I had other problems now. My light had gone out. Unlike the adult riders, who had brought along two bikes, I just had one and no replacement parts. A guy came riding by with his light burning bright. "Come on, kid, get on my wheel," he said. I never found out who he was but he helped lead me through the last two laps.

On the fourteenth lap, I passed a guy named John Moorhouse, who had been ahead of me for eleven and a half hours. That had to hurt, seeing this kid come by so late in the race with no light, and hanging on to someone else's wheel. But a half mile from the checkpoint, things suddenly went south for Southerland. My tire exploded, and I rode the flat into the pit area. I figured I was done, and that I'd sewn up second place. I had no desire to go out for another lap. But then Moorhouse came riding into the tent and his support crew started shouting to him, "The kid's light's dead! The kid's light's dead!" I remember he looked like I felt, half dead at that point and probably not thinking too clearly after nearly twelve hours on the bike.

"Huh?" he said.

"The kid's light's dead. He won't be allowed to continue. All you have to do is finish this lap and you get second place."

His crew replaced the battery pack, and with his light shining brightly he struggled out and continued riding. I remember saying to Jeff, "What the hell is going on?" An official came over to me. "You have no light, son, you can't go on, sorry." The thought of losing second place reenergized me. I pleaded with the official to let me continue. I'd memorized the course by now, so I didn't need a light, I told them. I could get on somebody's wheel and ride, just as I'd done the preceding lap. In desperation, I called out for an extra battery pack or a spare light, but no one in the tent either heard me or had anything to spare. I started to get upset. "That's not fair!" I shouted. But then Jeff put his hand on my shoulder. "Phil, you done good . . . damn good," he said in a soothing voice. "You don't want to get hurt now."

I started to think about it: I'd taken third place in one of the longest bike races ever held in the state of Florida. I was sixteen and a diabetic. *Damn,* I thought. *Jeff was right. I did good.*

Now, I was also starting to pay the price for having completed fourteen laps, or about ninety-six miles, on a mountain bike. There was a changing room and showers for us near the finish. I was caked in mud from head to toe at this point, so before we got back into Jeff's car and headed home, I wanted to get cleaned up. I sat down on the locker room bench, bent down to take my shoes off . . . and couldn't get up. My back had tightened up after twelve hours on the bike, and now I could not even sit up straight. It was a terrifying feeling, and I started to panic. "Hey, I need some help," I called out. "Someone . . . help!" Jeff had gone to the car, so he was out of earshot, but someone else came running in, helped me slowly straighten up, get my clothes off, and helped me stagger into the shower.

Late that night, we were back on a Florida highway, heading home. I sat in the backseat, cradling a trophy that was nearly as big as me. Around midnight, Jeff said to his girlfriend, "Helluva job, I'm proud of him." I fell asleep. I was dead tired.

As we drove along, the thought popped back into my mind: *Hey, I want my hundred bucks!* I'd forgotten about the bet during the race, but now the thought of a nice crisp C-note in my pocket was comforting. It took me a while, but eventually I did collect from Kenny Williams. I also earned something more important. At Revolutions, I noticed that I was being treated differently than I had in the three years since I first walked into the store with my mom. Sure, everybody still busted my hump—just like they did everyone else's—but I began to feel less like a mascot and more like a bike racer. I'd done something none of them ever had—raced twelve hours nonstop on a mountain bike. Now, instead of derisive laughter about the little jerk whose headlight went out, there was serious talk about how I'd been screwed out of second place on a technicality. Other riders started asking me my opinion about racing and riding. Nobody called me Philbert anymore (nobody, that is, except Ray, who *still* calls me Philbert). Looking back, my third-place trophy from the twelve-hour race was like an honors diploma. I'd graduated from being a kid pedaling around the neighborhood to a serious mountain-bike racer; from a boy to a young man. Now, I was about to leave for a new kind of school, a new kind of experience.

5

On the Road

In a bicycle race billed as the world's toughest something seems to be missing as riders converge here: FEAR. [For] RAAM racers, a certain calm and respect seems to be intermingled with their auras, like a boxer who knows his opponent is going to lay a beating on him for 10 or 12 rounds, but who still expects to endure and emerge through the pain to raise his arms in victory. This is the rational thought of man facing adversity. You need to have faith in your preparation, your crew, your equipment and most importantly yourself.

—RAAM BLOG

The twelve-hour race represented the pinnacle of my mountain-biking career. Yet, even as I ground my way around the Rock, I had already begun steering myself in a new direction as a cyclist. To explain how that happened, I need to back up our story here for a moment to April 1997—about nine months before the twelve-hour race. That's when I went for the first time to watch a race I would later know well: The Twilight Criterium in Athens, Georgia.

This was the first road cycling event I'd ever seen. As I was still a die-hard Revolutionary at that point, immersed in the daredevil world of the fat tire, I regarded this variation of the sport with the acidic disdain that only an adolescent can muster.

I went to Athens with Joel, the kid who was part of my J Gang plus P, which had first started riding listless loops of Tallahassee together a couple of summers earlier. We drove up with Jeff Asbell, one of the Revolutions guys. As mountain bikers, we were into showing attitude, especially in this fancy-ass college town, so the Friday night before the race, I shaved my hair into a Mohawk, died it red and green, and then poured Elmer's glue over the whole mess so that my single hedgerow of hairs stood up like bristles in a brush. Joel had coiffed himself in a similar style. Looking like refugees from a Sex Pistols concert, we wandered the streets of Athens, with Jeff—a fire hydrant of a guy—guarding us and glaring at any of the frat boys who made comments. "You got a problem with that?" he snarled to one beer-swilling group that laughed at the "redneck punks." Jeff was ex-military and you could tell it in his demeanor. They shut up. But we didn't. "Look at those dorks on the skinny tires," I laughed, as we saw the criterium competitors milling around before the start of the pro race. We were bad-ass mountain bikers, and if your tires weren't fat, you weren't cool in our book. And those outfits! Tights and pansy colors. "They look ridiculous," said Joel, as I nodded my red-and-green Elmer's-glued head in solemn agreement. "Yeah," I agreed. "A bunch of fags. And check out those bikes. My bike could kick their bikes' asses." We laughed hard and long at that one.

But when the race started, and those road dorks started whizzing by us at speeds unimaginable to a couple of punk mountain bikers, our attitudes softened—just slightly. *Huh,* I remember thinking. *They do go pretty fast.* I was also impressed by the prospect of a nice, bloody crash. We fell all the time in mountain biking, so we knew something about that, although falling on concrete, as the roadies did, made for a much gorier result than our tumbles on soft sand.

That night, I went home, sold my mountain bike, and became a die-hard roadie.

Not really.

When I got home that night, what really happened was that my mom saw what I'd done with my hair and flipped out. "You look like an idiot!" she screamed. "Why would you do that?"

I responded with the almost imperceptible shrug of the shoulders that parents of any adolescent will recognize as the universal gesture of teen cluelessness.

Not long after, I heard that Andy and Chris and some of the other mountain bikers were planning to do some road riding to help get them in better shape for the mountain-bike races. I couldn't call *these* guys—my friends—dorks, and I remembered how fast those riders had been going at Twilight. I began to reassess my views. If riding a road bike was going to help me get better as a mountain biker, maybe I ought to consider it. But a new sport meant new equipment—specifically, a new bike. A new bike that my mom was not going to be paying for, particularly since I was now at the charming teenage stage where most of my responses to her were in the form of grunts, and since I now spent more time at Revolutions or on the trails than I did at home.

In short, I needed money.

This was June, and on the last night of school, a Friday, I was over at the Costigans' for a party. My mom, Sheila, and the other adults were upstairs, drinking wine. The "young-uns" were outside shooting hoops and playing ping-pong. One of them was a friend of mine called W.J., whose dad, Jerome Cox, owned a successful door-products business in Tallahassee. I had an idea.

"Hey, man," I said to W.J., "I could use a job this summer. You think I could get some work with your dad?"

"Dunno," he said. "Ask him."

Normally, that would have been enough to have kept me seated on the couch. I was still a shy kid and I was secretly hoping that W.J. would ask his dad for me. But that night, my desire for cash prompted me to take action. I screwed up my courage, walked upstairs, and found Mr. Cox chatting with a few of the other parents, wineglasses in hand. I walked right up to him.

"Excuse, me, Mr. Cox," I said.

"Hey, Phil, what's up?"

I took a breath and then asked the question: "Well, sir, I was wondering if you might need any help at the store this summer?"

I was fifteen and a half, so it was a borderline call, because you had to be sixteen to get working papers. But I think Mr. Cox liked the fact that I had asked him directly and politely.

"Sure, I think we can find something for you, provided you show up on time and work hard."

"I certainly will, sir," I said as earnestly as if I were swearing a blood oath. "I'll work as hard as anybody."

He chuckled. "I think you will, son. When can you start?"

This was Friday. Monday was the first day of summer vacation.

"Monday, sir. If that's good with you."

"Monday it is, Phil. Look forward to having you onboard."

I shook his hand, somewhat incredulous.

That's all it took, I thought to myself. *I just had to ask.* It was an important lesson I would remember in the future, when what I was asking for added up to significantly more than I'd be making with Mr. Cox—$5.15 an hour. But at fifteen, those wages looked mighty fine to me. On Monday at 7:30 A.M., while most of my friends were still fast asleep on the first day of vacation, I started my first job.

Working in Mr. Cox's door business, I learned that when you sell a door, you sell the frame that comes with it and the bolts that go with the frame. Jerome Cox sold a lot of doors: we'd get in huge orders from office buildings or factories that were being built or renovated, and part of my job was to help organize the doors based on height and weight. I'd work with the seasoned vets in the warehouse, who would give me directions on how to sort them, and I spent many a morning that summer huffing and puffing as I pushed and pulled the doors into neat piles, ready for delivery. As the days went on, I'd go on the deliveries and help with the installations. I'd also sweep out the warehouse, run errands, do any little thing that was needed.

There was plenty to do, and if I worked more than forty hours, Jerome said, he'd pay me overtime. So I tried to put in as many hours as possible, often working ten hours a day. It added up. When I got my first paycheck, I had my mom drive me right over to Revolutions, where I bought a used road bike for four hundred dollars. The bike had belonged to Jeff Sukach, one of the shorter adult riders among the Revolutions crew, and Chris figured it would be the perfect frame for little ol' me. He was right.

My new road bike became my primary mode of transportation. Every morning at seven, I'd hop on and ride the six miles to the store. There, I'd change out of my bike outfit, put on my Door Products uniform, punch the clock, and start sweeping or stocking or unloading and stacking the doors. It was hard work, especially in that warehouse, where the torrid summer temperatures sometimes reached 110 degrees. Worse than the heat was the country music blasting on the speakers set up in the rafters. The good ol' boys who ran the warehouse would hear of nothing else and called me a hippie or a freak when I had the temerity to suggest we put on some rock-and-roll. As much as they poked fun of me—my bike outfits, as well as my musical preferences, were a particular target—I came to like the guys in the warehouse. They were all in their twenties and thirties, and they were stereotypical rebels. They loved their guns, their girls, their pickup trucks, and their cold Buds on hot summer nights—very different from most of the kids I'd grown up around in Piedmont Park; very different from the adults I was riding bikes with.

But as much as they were good ol' boys, they were also good men: hard workers, loyal to Mr. Cox, in large part because he treated them fairly. They were conscientious and honest, and in their own way they watched out for me. I found that out during one of the red-letter days of that summer, and of every adolescent boy's life: the first time I got blistering drunk.

It happened at Mr. Cox's house, which in retrospect was exceptionally stupid, considering that he was my employer. He was away for the day, and his son W.J. had the place to himself. So he gathered about four of his friends together and broke out the booze. We drank rum and Coke. I think we also drank scotch and Coke. Maybe vodka and Coke, too. End result: I got annihilated, puked all over the nice rug in W.J.'s bedroom, and my friends had to help walk me home.

This classy soiree was on a Thursday. I stayed over at W.J.'s house that night and somehow stumbled into work the next morning, where I very quickly threw up again. I was dizzy, a mess, and I finally had to go to Mr. Cox to tell him I was too sick to work. I called my mom and she arrived, angry as a rattlesnake. She knew what was going on as soon as she saw me. "You got drunk last night, didn't you?" she said, as I stood pale and wobbly in front of her. At that point, Trent, one of the warehouse guys, spoke up. "Mrs. Southerland," he drawled in a contrite tone, "it's not his fault. You see, some of us, we took him out last night and . . . well, I know it was wrong, but we kept him out a little too late. So you see, it's really that the boy is just *tired*—"

Joanna threw a sharp glance his way, stopping him in midsentence. "Yeah, right." Then she turned back to me. "Let's go, Phil." I turned around to see Trent shrugging his shoulders, a sympathetic "I tried my best" expression on his face. I nodded wearily, because I knew what was to come. The wrath of Joanna.

"You *did* get drunk last night, didn't you?" she said.

"No, I didn't."

"That's a load of bull and you know it. What did you drink? Tell me, or you're going to be grounded for the rest of the summer."

Pause, sigh, and a moan.

"Okay . . . I drank rum and scotch."

She shook her head incredulously. Not only was I an underage drinker, I was an underage drinker who didn't have a clue about how to mix his drinks.

"You are a dumbass," she concluded. "And when we get home, you're mowing the lawn."

That was a stiff sentence, as I hated mowing the lawn under the best of circumstances, and these were hardly the best of circumstances. I felt like crap and it was one of the hottest days of the summer. The heat index in Tallahassee that day was 115. There I was, trying to mow our lawn while nursing one of the great hangovers in human history. I'd push the mower across one strip of grass, stop, and puke. Then I'd push it across another strip, stop, and puke. It went on for hours like that and I can only imagine what the neighbors thought.

What did I gain from this experience? Well, it's been thirteen years and I still haven't touched another drop of scotch. I also learned something about drinking for diabetics, candid advice I often pass along to young adults with type 1. Parents and doctors will say simply, *Don't drink*. And if you choose not to, that's great. But I'm realistic, so I know that most adolescents experiment with alcohol at some point. If so, use your head. Remember that depending on what you drink, alcohol will often cause a temporary elevation of your blood sugar, and then later it'll come crashing down. Make sure your friends know what to do when that happens. I would tell my buddies when we'd go out for drinks, "If I start acting any dumber than I normally do, it probably means my blood sugar is low. So get me a Gatorade or some sugar."

As for my first disastrous foray into drinking, I learned the importance not only of drinking responsibly but of taking responsibility. I should have owned up to it right away. While I appreciated what Trent tried to do, covering for me in front of my mom, I'd made a stupid mistake and had to face the music.

At least it wasn't country-and-western.

Every Saturday, as part of their road training, the Revolutions guys and other local bike racers gathered together for a group ride that began in the parking lot of what used to be a Food Lion supermarket in Tallahassee. While admittedly not as famous as the annual Florida State–Florida football game, the Saturday-morning Food Lion ride, as it was known, was a long-running Tally tradition, starting back in the 1970s. About thirty to forty riders would gather in the parking lot and head out on a thirty-two-mile road course that would wind its way through the outer suburbs of the city and on into the countryside.

That summer, Chris and some of the guys invited me to come along on my new road bike. This was considered an honor, and it came with all kinds of caveats. "The Food Lion ride is really hard and really competitive, so don't worry if you can't hang on," Chris said, probably remembering my first time out on a mountain-bike ride with him and the group. "We'll come back and get you."

But I wasn't the same kid who had been dropped like a rock two years earlier. I was leaner and stronger. Racing had given me confidence on the bike. I listened and nodded to all the well-intentioned warnings about how difficult it would be to stay up with the Food Lion group, and on my first ride I finished with the leaders. "Nice job," they said. "Good going, kid."

"Yeah, thanks," I replied, trying to act as bored and nonchalant as possible. Inside, though, I was thrilled. The twelve-hour race had given me confidence. I was tired of being seen as the Revolutions mascot. Besides, by that point, I was starting to develop into a decent sprinter. Working in the warehouse that summer, riding my bike to and from work, the long training rides, all had helped me lose about twenty pounds off my already small frame. While Joanna complained that I looked emaciated, I felt razor-sharp fit. I started to get more aggressive on the group rides, which soon included not only the Food Lion on Saturday but other group-training rides during the week. I would strike without warning, taking the rest of the group by surprise in a sudden surge to the front. Maybe it was because I was juiced up with adolescent type 1 anger and an overpowering urge to prove myself. Maybe it was just because I was tired of being looked at as "the kid" by the other riders. Maybe it was dawning on me that my life was going to take me away from Tallahassee and so I'd better start moving.

Whatever the reason, I did start riding faster, started getting more competitive. I would eventually win the Junior State Championships that summer. I began challenging Andy during flat stretches of the Food Lion ride. We'd run our mouths as we sprinted alongside each other (I was becoming a grade-A trash talker). Soon, Andy recalls, "it became a personal battle between Phil and me. We wouldn't worry about the rest of the group. As long as I beat him, it would be fine."

In retrospect, I'm not sure which is more incredible—that there was such a thing as a diabetic cycling camp or that I actually agreed to attend.

I thought I was such hot stuff cycling at this point, riding with guys twice my age, that I'm sure I must have sneered at the very idea of going to a camp with a bunch of kids. I was already fifteen by now, a little old for camp, but when I got the opportunity, and Mom was willing to pay for it, I thought, *What the heck?* I'd made decent money that summer. So why not?

Diabetes camps weren't common then, much less one devoted to a sport. But the diabetes cycling camp I attended in Gainesville, Florida that summer was a pretty good idea—ahead of its time, I think, as I look back.

I had done a thirty-mile race that morning, and my mom drove me from there right to the camp. "He's had a really active day already," she told the counselor, as I went off to play a game of touch football. As I recall, that was just the beginning of a busy afternoon of sports. It was fun—but the next morning, when they had a tough time rousing me out of my sleep, everyone just assumed that I was another slug teenager who liked to sleep until noon.

The truth was that with that much activity, I should have reduced my insulin, which didn't happen. No one thought that I might be hypoglycemic and that the thing I really needed wasn't sleep, but food. When I finally got myself up, I stumbled out of my tent and over to the mess tent. One minute I'm waiting there with my tray in hand, and starting to tell myself that I don't feel well . . . and the next minute I'm waking up in a hospital. Ironic: my first seizure in many years, and it happens at a diabetic bicycling camp!

They weren't happy about it and my mom wasn't happy with them—she figured they should have been more on top of it—but in the end it all worked out. I had a great week at camp. I also had a crush on the prettiest girl in there. She, on the other hand, had not the slightest interest in the shortest guy in camp—me—even though most of the other campers were impressed with my riding skills. This after all wasn't really a camp for developing high-level competitive-racing skills. It was basically a place where adolescent diabetics could come and meet other adolescents with diabetes—and in the process have a lot of fun, a week sleeping in tents and who knows what else. The bike riding was almost incidental.

I did learn something that would help me better understand my fellow diabetics. Unlike most of the kids in that camp, I had never known anything but being type 1. These kids had. Many of them had just been diagnosed in the preceding few years, and they were bitter and confused about it all. They went to this camp, in part, to feel normal—to feel like they weren't pariahs or outcasts because of a disease that had suddenly, and without any fault of their own, irrevocably changed their lives. I realized that in a way, being diagnosed at seven months, had been a blessing. And I wouldn't take that for granted in the future, when I started inter-acting more with other people with type 1.

I came back from camp in time to put in a few more days of work at the door-products warehouse. The Friday before Labor Day weekend, I laid my last door on a palette for Mr. Cox. "Get the hell out of my shop!" he said as I came in to wish him good-bye. Then he laughed, and he put his arm around me. "Phil, you're a good kid. We enjoyed having you here this summer."

I enjoyed being there—well, maybe not enough that I wanted to quit school and work the rest of my life in a 110-degree warehouse. I had thrived on the structured regimen of work and training. The thought of going back to high school was depressing—but, I had to admit, only slightly more depressing than the idea of working in that warehouse the rest of my life. Don't get me wrong, I really liked Trent and the other good ol' boys in the warehouse, even though they called me a spandex-wearing wuss and said that if I loved bike riding so much I ought to move to "Frantz" or go live with the *Eye*talians. All that ball busting aside, they were solid fellows with good hearts, who'd do anything for you. I think they brought out a little more of the South in Southerland.

Problem was, I didn't want to do what they were doing for the rest of my life. In order to avoid a life spent in a warehouse . . . *any* warehouse . . . I'd have to go to college, and to get to college I'd have to make decent grades in high school. So, that fall, I finally hunkered down at Leon High. But I was still shy, suspicious, and gripped by a sense of insecurity that was a direct result of being the shortest kid in my class and the second-to-last male to have gone through puberty (such things were carefully noticed and tracked in the boys' locker room during gym class).

It's funny: here I was able to mouth off to hirsute rednecks with tattoos, walk up to a prominent local businessman and bluntly ask for a job, and exchange barbs with a cluster of six-foot-tall guys in their thirties while racing bicycles—but the prospect of talking to a sixteen-year-old made me break out in a cold sweat. I simply didn't know how to have conversations with my peers. Throw me in a room—or preferably on a bike trail—with a bunch of guys twice my age and I could trash talk all morning. But among adolescents, male and female, I was always worried about what people were thinking, always concerned about what I should say. So, typically, in and around Leon High I said nothing. I had a small circle of friends, but by and large it was an empty place for me.

That winter, I trained for my Ocala twelve-hour race. Almost immediately afterward, though, my bike riding took on a new direction.

It was in Gainesville, March 1998, just seven days after the twelve-hour ride in Ocala. A guy named Ace Lashley—then one of the better riders in Tallahassee—had heard about my grit in the twelve-hour and invited me to attend a race with him. He was older, a good cyclist, and I was flattered. I said yes immediately, even though I had no idea what to do. That morning, Ace had to show me some of the most basic aspects of bike racing on the roads, such as where to pin your race number. In a mountain-bike race, you attach it to your bike. In a road you pin your number to your jersey. (Thanks, Ace, for preventing me from making a total fool of myself!) My complete ignorance about road racing, however, didn't dampen my confidence or my cockiness. I rolled up to the start line of the juniors' race, figuring that since I'd just done an ultradistance race, I was probably a lot stronger than most of these guys. I'd simply outlast them and then, at the end, stun them all with a devastating Food Lion–like attack.

What I didn't understand is that in road racing, there are tactics far more complex and often more subtle than in mountain biking or even on group rides. I was now part of the rolling chess game that is road cycling, but in terms of my understanding of it all, I might as well have been playing Go Fish. Off we went, on a twenty-five-mile course laid out in a triangle shape. I just followed the wheels ahead of me, knowing that I had the strength to keep up, believing I had the speed to make a big move at the end. We get to the last turn. The finish line, I thought, was about two hundred yards away. I attack, and despite the fact that I'm slipping in and out of the mountain-bike pedals that I had on my road bike, I'm ahead of everybody else. My first road race and I'm going to win! This was going to be even easier than I'd thought.

Not so fast, Phil. I had misjudged the distance. It was probably more like 350 to 400 yards left to go to the finish when we'd made that turn. Very few racers can hold a flat-out sprint for that long. I felt myself faltering, and just then . . . two guys who had correctly judged the distance, and timed their attack better than I did, went flying by. Race over, I was third. "Son of a bitch!" I gasped, as I rolled to a stop. The guy who'd finished first glanced over with a smirk on his face. I just scowled back. He was Daniel Holt, one of the top junior racers in Florida. Although he would later become one of my best friends, I hated his guts that day, for being smarter and faster and more experienced than I was.

There *was* a small consolation prize: I'd won a whopping twenty dollars for finishing third. Driving back with Ace—who'd finished in sixth place in the pro race—we celebrated with a big pig-out at Waffle House.

Money was still on my mind at this point. I was now sixteen, and that meant I could get working papers and take an on-the-books job. My mom was still working hard to make ends meet and I knew I'd need money to support my bike habit and, eventually, to get a car, take girls out on dates, and do some of the other stuff that adolescents did (even though I wasn't doing any of them yet). That spring, after the twelve-hour race and my rude awakening in the Gainesville road race, I got a job at the Publix supermarket on Thomasville Road in Tallahassee, bagging groceries.

That something as pedestrian as filling other people's shopping bags with boxes of cornflakes and quarts of milk could register as a decisive point in my or anyone's life might sound ridiculous. But I can honestly tell you: I learned more about life there, more about people, more about business management, more about myself than I did in four years of high school. Part of the reason that Publix provided such an excellent education is the company's philosophy. This chain of supermarkets in the Southeast has a mission-and-values statement that their management has actually read, and believes in. Check it out:

At Publix, we commit to be:

- Passionately focused on Customer Value,
- Intolerant of Waste,
- Dedicated to the Dignity, Value and Employment Security of our Associates,
- Devoted to the highest standards of stewardship for our Stockholders, and
- Involved as Responsible Citizens in our Communities

They really believe this. Just as important, they've been damn successful doing business this way. For the last fifteen years, Publix has made *Fortune*'s list of both the Most Admired Companies and the Best Companies to Work For in the United States. Their customer-approval ratings are off the charts, and *Business Week* listed them as one of their Customer Service Champs among U.S. companies. (And trust me, I'm not a paid Publix spokesperson or anything like that. It's been years since I worked there.)

You don't get that kind of reputation by being inefficient and inattentive. From day one, I was schooled in the science of grocery bagging (I bet you didn't know there *was* a science). We learned to work fast and efficiently, to keep the lines from backing up. We'd fill each bag with as many items as possible to save plastic and paper, but do so carefully to keep anything from getting crushed. We were taught to keep cold with cold, hot with hot, dry with dry. Fitting various-shaped boxes into the same bag almost became fun—like a little geometry puzzle. (Maybe it's not surprising that around this time, geometry became my best subject.) Then we would carry the bags out to the customer's car. Because Publix didn't want surly, incommunicative teenagers accompanying chatty, little old ladies to the parking lot, the company encouraged polite talk with the customers while you were assisting them. At first I was terrified over the prospect of chitchatting with people I didn't know. But then I realized that this was an opportunity to improve my social skills, frustrated as I was with my insecure high-school self. So I began to use the job as a way to learn and practice the art of small talk. I figured out that about every eight minutes, I was carrying a new person's groceries out to his or her car. Over my four-hour shift, that was a total of twenty-eight opportunities for conversation with different individuals. I listened to some of the other baggers and practiced different methods of greeting.

"Hey" sounded too casual.

"Wassup?" was too gen X, too hip-hop.

"Good afternoon, ma'am"—too southern and stilted.

Eventually, I found that "How are *you* today?" worked best. It put the spotlight on the customers and got them to talk about the most important thing in their lives: themselves. It also signaled that I cared—and I really tried to care. My bag-carrying conversations taught me to listen as much as talk, and listen I did. While it would be titillating to report that people confessed their darkest secrets and poured their hearts out to the friendly Publix bag boy, it was mostly small talk. But as time went by, I did get to know some of the regulars by name. I knew their families, knew what they did; and in turn they'd ask me about school and bike racing. We also had a couple of celebrities come into our store: once, I bagged groceries for Brad Johnson, a former Florida State star who lived in Tallahassee and was then playing quarterback for the Minnesota Vikings (I don't remember much except that he had a lot of groceries, not surprising considering he was six feet five inches, 238 pounds).

We also had a guy from the alt-rock band Creed come in once. The others baggers were too scared to go up to him, so I did. "How are *you* today?" He kind of grunted, as I recall. When I went to take his bags out, he said, "No, no, I'll do it." I told him it was my pleasure. "No, thanks," he said firmly. "I want to do it."

"Look, if I don't carry your bags, I'm going to get fired." So the rock-and-roll millionaire finally let me carry his groceries out to the car.

A pro football player and a rock star could have afforded to give me a tip, but we weren't allowed to accept them. That was the rule: no gratuities. But after a while, some of the Publix veterans took me aside and told me that if a customer offered me a dollar or two, I should just take it. As my social skills improved, I found that if I took customers' groceries out to the parking lot, put the bags in their trunks, chatted with them about the weather or school or whatever, they'd almost invariably reach into the pocket or the purse and hand over a couple of dollars, a dollar, even a handful of change. All donations were gladly accepted, and as I honed my interpersonal skills, the tips started rolling in. It was working beautifully until one day a Publix manager caught me counting a wad of bills (since they were mostly singles, it probably didn't amount to much, but looked thick enough to catch his eye).

"Son, where'd you get that?" he asked suspiciously.

"Uh . . ."

"It's tip money, isn't it?"

"No, sir, no it isn't."

"You know our rules about tips, don't you?"

"I do, sir. But let me put it to you this way: wouldn't you find it insulting if someone refused your gratitude?"

"What do you mean?"

"I take the time to talk to our customers, find out how they're doing. I get to know them."

"That's good, that's what we want you to do."

"Right, so when these folks offer me a couple of dollars, and I refuse it, it's almost insulting to them. They're showing *their* loyalty and appreciation to us by offering that money, and so by refusing it *we're* kind of being disloyal to them, if you see what I mean."

He paused and processed the argument that, to my surprise, had somehow formed and rolled off my tongue as smoothly as if I'd rehearsed it for days.

"Well, when you present it that way, okay. Just don't go asking for tips."

"I certainly won't, sir."

That day, I learned that I could now do more than engage in small talk. I could think on my feet and talk my way out of a tight situation. I hesitate to say that I realized that day I was a good bullshitter, so put it this way: it was then and there that I decided that maybe if I couldn't ride a bike for a living, maybe my career should be in sales. Exactly what I would sell, I couldn't yet foresee, but I certainly never thought it would have anything to do with the disease that I was pedaling away from as fast as I could.

That summer before my junior year in high school, a guy named Louis LaMarche popped up on the Tally bike-racing scene. This was news at Revolutions and on the Food Lion ride. LaMarche was probably the best bike racer to have come out of Tallahassee to that point. He was Ace Lashley times five: a guy who as a junior racer had finished fourth in the national championship. He'd even raced in Europe for a couple of years. However, he had contracted spinal meningitis and had to stop competing, and was now making a comeback.

With my newfound confidence, I had no trouble going up to LaMarche and telling him I wanted to learn everything I could from him. I was now determined to become a competitive road cyclist—those skinny tires no longer looked as dorky as they had to me a year or two earlier—and I knew that the only way to *get* better was to ride with people who *were* better. I tried to stay on Louis's wheel all summer on the rides, watching how he positioned himself and how he attacked. It was the beginning of a year-long education that would have as big an impact on my riding as my job in Publix had on my interpersonal skills.

Through the summer, fall, and into the winter of 1999, I did most of my training with Louis and Ray. On the weekends there were training criterium races in Tampa, and Louis suggested we drive down there. You'd sign up, pay seven dollars, and compete in an hour-long race on a criterium (closed) course. On the drive down to the first of these crits, Louis taught me about the racing mind-set. "If you're scared, you're going to lose, Phil," he explained. "And what we're most afraid of is the pain. So when it's five laps to go, you've just got to turn the 'fear' switch off. The race is almost over, the finish line is practically there, and at that point you just need to put the pain aside. You've earned the finish at this point, you can't let your fear of hurting stand in your way."

I listened intently. He was right—I was afraid of pain. Who isn't? It's almost unnatural to ignore discomfort, to keep going when your body says, *Stop, this hurts!* That's what sets competitive athletes apart, especially in endurance sports like bicycling and running, where the pain is not sharp and momentary but long and burning and unrelenting, like a fire rising from your legs that eventually spreads across your entire body, so that you can feel you're being burned alive. That's pain—and *that,* Louis was saying, was what a good racing cyclist learns to ignore, even to master.

I tried to put the lessons Louis had taught me to the test. Remembering how I'd been burned in my first road race in Gainesville, I stayed patient in that first crit, and hung with the pack. Because it was a training race, all the racers at every level were riding together—as opposed to the different age and ability "cats," or categories—so I could see Louis ahead of me and tried to mimic everything he was doing. When he relaxed, I relaxed; when he attacked, I attacked. When he stayed cool even though I knew he must be hurting, I tried to stay cool, remembering the "no fear" attitude he had encouraged me to adopt. At the end, in the big field sprint—when the entire field pedals like mad for the finish line— I hammered, and finished two places behind the great Louis LaMarche. Granted, this was a training race; admittedly, he was in comeback mode, but for me it was pretty damn awesome.

However, just to make certain I didn't get a swelled head, Louis and Ray decided to burst my bubble—or maybe my bladder. After the race, we hit a convenience store before getting on the highway home. I bought a supersize, sixty-four-ounce Diet Coke. "Don't drink that, Phil," Ray said. "You'll have to pee, and we ain't stopping." I ignored him and chugged the whole thing down. Sure enough, as we were cruising up I-75 a half hour later, I had to use the bathroom. "Nope!" said Ray, who was driving, as Louis chuckled. "We warned you." So I had to sit in the damn car for two and a half hours before they finally agreed to pull over at a Dairy Queen.

The message was clear: you're a still a punk kid. So when we tell you something, listen.

That trip established a template for that winter. Every weekend we'd head out of Tally on I-10 east to to I-75 south, and take that down to Tampa—a four-hour drive. We'd eat in the cheapest restaurant, crash at the cheapest motel we could find, then get up the morning, race the crit, and head home. On the way back we'd always stop at that same Dairy Queen off exit 37 on I-10. The first time I went in there to eat (as opposed to using their bathroom), I did five units of insulin to compensate for the large Oreo Blizzard I intended to devour. It seemed worth every bite, until I checked my blood sugar an hour and a half later: It was 350. Now here comes decision time. A lot of people with diabetes would have said, "Okay, that's it. No more Oreo Blizzards for me." But, perhaps because that Blizzard was *sooooo* good, and I was a teenager who didn't want to be denied any pleasure, I tried to look at it from a different perspective:

Maybe the problem wasn't the food. Maybe the problem was that I hadn't done enough insulin before indulging in the food.

The next weekend, we headed down to Tampa again for another crit. I had another good race, and to celebrate, Louis, Ray, and I went back to the same Dairy Queen on the way home. The weekend before, I'd taken five units of insulin. So this time I did seven, and when I checked my blood sugar later, it was 50 . . . too low. I'd done a little too much. The following week, I got it just right, with six units of insulin leading to one more delicious dessert.

As with alcohol, I'm not saying here that diabetics should go hog wild at Dairy Queen or on any other type of dessert. But you don't always have to say, "I can't eat this." It may be more a question of *how* you eat than what you eat—or, more specifically, how you manage your insulin and blood sugar around your eating.

I'd learned that successful bike racing was about experiment-
ing, making mistakes, and trying to improve the next time. Diabetes, I came to realize, was the same game: learning from the
mistakes I made today and trying not to make them tomorrow.

As far as I could tell, I was the only one enjoying the fruits of
this education because I didn't know any other diabetic that raced
bicycles. I suppose if I had searched I could have found some other
type 1 who was riding. But I wasn't looking to become part of the
larger diabetes community at this point, in part because there really wasn't one. There was the American Diabetes Association, sure,
and I suppose there were some support groups, but for the most
part, diabetics tended to be on their own. Outside of your family, it
was just you and your endocrinologist. What we were hearing
wasn't very encouraging. It was always about what you couldn't or
shouldn't do.

You can't do this . . . you shouldn't do that . . . don't let this happen . . .
you better not get to this point . . . on and on, all of it a message of
"not." I'm sure that most endocrinologists in the late 1990s would
have told me you better *not* keep training like that, you probably
shouldn't be bike racing, and, oh no, you *can't* be eating those Oreo
Blizzards.

Fortunately, no doc ever did, in part because with my bike-punk
attitude at that point, I would have probably flipped 'em the bird
and walked out of his office. Lucky for me, though, I had a pediatric endocrinologist who was more forward-thinking than most in
her profession at the time. Her name was Nancy Wright, and she
took over my care in 1997. Dr. Wright—or Nancy, as I have come to
know her—was a bike rider herself, so she encouraged all her patients to engage in exercise and sports. I liked her from the start, in
part because she was interested in more than my blood sugar. She
liked to talk about training, bikes, and other aspects of my life, as

well as my diabetes. During my quarterly checkups with her, I began to feel that she was a collaborator, a partner, someone interested in helping me achieve my goal of becoming a better bike racer while controlling my diabetes. Most remarkably, she listened carefully and appreciatively when I told her about my efforts to control my disease (à la my Dairy Queen experiments), and sometimes it seemed she was learning from me. Quite amazing to a teenager that an adult would find anything you had to say edifying, but that's Nancy's philosophy to this day. "Young people with type 1 diabetes *are* experts on their disease," she says. "They're the ones who live with it each day."

For Nancy, I think I was an interesting patient because I had such a severe case of type 1. She had never heard of anyone diagnosed as young as I; by that point, I really didn't have a pancreas, and yet there I was, blasting around on a racing bike. "Phil and I strategized a lot about how to keep his diabetes in control, about how to maximize his bike performance without having severe low blood sugar," Nancy recalls. At the time there were newer forms of insulin coming out; Nancy introduced these to me, and they helped my control to become even more precise. Besides her obvious intelligence and professionalism, I also just liked *her*—she was younger than most of the docs I'd dealt with, she had a great personality, and the fact that she was a bicyclist was a bonus. I'd actually see her sometimes when I was out riding, which was cool. She tells a funny story about that.

"I was riding with a few friends through the Munson Hills one weekend," Nancy says. "All of a sudden, here come these three riders from the other direction, going really fast. They just blew right past us. We had to get out of the way. As they whizzed by, I heard one of them yell to the other, 'Hey, be careful, that's my doctor!' He turned around and gave me a big grin, and I saw it was Phil."

Although I didn't recognize it at the time, the arrival of endo-crinologists like Nancy, progressive health professionals who took a positive, can-do approach to what those with type 1 could do, was changing the diabetes world. While I didn't yet see myself as some-one who would be part of that change—I was still just a type 1 kid learning his way in life and in his sport—I'm sure that my interac-tions with Nancy in those years helped plant a seed that would flower a few years later.

At the time of this writing, Dr. Wright is still practicing in Tal-lahassee, still helping type 1 kids and their families. When those patients have a seat in her office, they see a framed, signed photo of me on my bike. Nancy calls me "a role model," which is generous and very humbling to hear today. But at the point we first started working together, my focus was still on becoming a cyclist worthy of that kind of honor. That was my goal—or maybe *obsession* would be a better word—as I went into the last two years of high school.

6

Snowman Lights a Fire

The sport is expensive, dangerous, time-consuming, mentally draining, emotionally exhausting and physically demanding and it permeates every aspect of a Roadie's life. I would describe it as a chess game, boxing match and stampede disguised as a sport encompassed by a lifestyle surrounded by a community on a never-ending road trip to the brink of bankruptcy. One can dabble in tennis, golf, softball, basketball and other sports. There is no dabbling in bike racing.

—JAMIE SMITH, *Roadie: The Misunderstood World of a Bike Racer*

I'm not a dabbler. I am about full-bore commitment to the point of pigheadedness. So when I took to the roads in my last two years in high school, it was in the almost obsessive way that Smith describes: with an absolute burning, fueled in part by all the torments typical to most adolescents, and no doubt in larger part by the realization that I was still what I had always been: small, fatherless, and diabetic.

Fortunately, and perhaps this is one reason why the sport appealed to me, bike racing didn't allow me the time to sit around and brood about my lot in life or my stature. While I may have been a pain in the ass to my mom during my teenage years, she certainly never had to worry about me hanging out with the "wrong crowd" (as some of my friends from childhood were already starting to do) or being lured into the temptations of narcotics, or alcohol, or even petty crime.

I had found my crowd and I had found my drug.

Every weekend during that winter and early spring of 1999—peak racing season in Florida—I would pile into the car with Ray and Louis LaMarche and drive four hours through the heart of the Sunshine State in order to race in circles in Tampa, as part of their winter criterium series, as well as races in Gainesville, Jacksonville, and elsewhere. The competition was keen: not only was there a lot of homegrown talent, you'd always get a lot of top guys from other, colder parts of the country, who would come down here to get some speed in their legs and competition at a time of year when there was ice and snow on the roads where they lived.

The events usually consisted of four or five separate races based on the proficiency categories (cats), staring with 5 for novices and descending to cats 4, 3, 2 and 1—which is where Louis was. There were also the juniors' (eighteen and under) races, which I often competed in, as well as occasional races where different levels and ages raced together.

Whatever and wherever the setup on a given weekend, I competed as much as I could, sometimes twice a day. I worked, I watched, I listened, I mouthed off, too, but I learned. My improvements became noticeable. I felt stronger and smoother on the bike, but just as important, I began to develop a better sense of what was going on around me in a race. Thanks to Louis, I began to learn how to read the peloton, understand the tactics, anticipate the moves. My results improved accordingly. I started creeping up in the finish places.

One weekend, I raced four times. In the morning I took eighth place in a cat 4 race and then that afternoon nailed another top-10 finish in a one-hundred-mile race I had impulsively jumped into. That's a lot of racing for one day, but the next morning—after a night of six of us crammed into a cheap motel room—I bounced back with seventeen-year-old resiliency, *won* the juniors' race (the first time I'd crossed a finish line in first place), and that afternoon I culminated the weekend by finishing third in another race, thanks to a hellacious push in the field sprint.

Four races, four top-ten finishes.

I felt like a stud, until after the last race, when I walked to the parking lot with Ray and Louis Lamarche.

"You did well," Louis said. "Now get in the car."

"Yeah," Ray chimed in. "And we're not stopping to pee, either."

I just rolled my eyes. They were right, of course. Louis that day had finished in the top five in the marquee pro event. There's a large hierarchy in cycling and I was still way down near the bottom.

My breakout weekend came the first weekend in March 1999, when I lined up for a cat 4 race in Jacksonville. That day, there was no separate competition for the juniors as there typically was during the winter events. The weather was cold—it may even have dipped into the high thirties—and this was a forty-mile road race on a circuit of rolling hills. To make matters more complicated, it started to rain—a cold, winter rain—during the first lap.

Precipitation always brings out the best—and worst—in a bike race. Some racers get totally turned on by bad weather: it motivates them to work harder. Others find it completely dispiriting: they slow down, whine, and basically throw in the towel. Either way, you have to be careful, alert, on your toes, because the already low margin of error between you racing upright on a bike and you splattered on the asphalt gets reduced to almost nothing on a slick road packed with guys going twenty-five miles per hour.

The possibility of a crash didn't faze me. Hell, I was a teenager, I'd crashed before, licked my wounds. What's the big deal? I rode confidently up to the front and, with three miles left, got on the wheel of the leader, a guy who had won most of the cat 4 races that year. I knew he was good, so I intended to stick with him. I was also aware that the other riders around me—all of them taller, older, more experienced—seemed noticeably tense. Gloves gripped the handlebars; faces were not only contorted with effort but creased with concern, like the expression of someone who just got a notice from the IRS in the mail. I realized why: these guys, and I knew most of them at least casually by now, all had jobs and careers and, in some cases, families to go back to the next morning. They had a lot to risk. A fall could mean days off from work, an angry spouse, chores left undone, medical bills to pay. For me, a broken collarbone would mean a couple of days home from school—hardly a penalty—and a badge of honor among my cycling buddies. My lips curled into an almost evil leer as I realized this.

"I'm not afraid to crash!" I said to the tight knot of cyclists around me. "Are you?"

One guy shot me an angry glance. That was the answer I needed. *Hasta la vista,* baby.

I annihilated the field sprint. When the leader—doubtless another member of the employed, responsible class—faltered with two hundred yards to go, I jumped him, flying by to win the race by a mile. And I mean that almost literally. I didn't see the finish line and just kept sprinting for another couple of hundred yards. I was shaking and blue from the cold at that point, but I was overjoyed. For me, a seventeen-year-old junior, to win a race against all these bigger, stronger, older—okay, and employed—adults, was the biggest moment of my racing life. I remember a lot of congratulations, a lot of high fives.

"Man, you killed those guys," said Louis. "Time to upgrade."

I knew exactly what he meant. With my hands shaking and cramped, I wrote down my ten best results of that season on a piece of soggy notepaper and walked straight over to E. J. Rogut, the top bike-racing official in Florida, who was getting ready for the pro race.

"M-mister Rogut, sir," I said, my teeth chattering, "I-I-I'd like you to look these over."

He took the paper and squinted at it through the rain.

"All right," he said, fishing a sticker out of his pocket. "You're a cat 3. Now go get into some dry clothes."

That was it: bike racing's equivalent of a battlefield promotion. By affixing that sticker to my USA Cycling bike-racing license, I had just advanced one major step up the hierarchy. I retreated to Ray's car feeling very satisfied. The next day, I won the juniors' race *and* finished in eighth place in my first race as a cat 3 rider.

Of course, throughout this time I was still a high school student, still working, and still a diabetic. And while I thought I was managing that as well as I was starting to handle my life as a bike racer slash Publix employee slash mediocre student, there were occasional scary moments.

One day when I was in study hall, we had the computers on to do our homework. I remember going into the classroom that day and staring into the computer. That's all I remember. The bell rang; it was time for Spanish class. Normally, I'd wait for these two girls who were in that study hall and we'd go to that class together. This time, I got up from the computer and walked out of the class, vacant-eyed, without a word. I went into the Spanish class and sat down at my desk. I was seated next to Jane, one of my friends. She had taken a candy bar and put it on her desk, I pointed at the bar and said, "Whatchamacallit"—the brand name of the candy. "Phil," she said, "you're a mooch. Get your own candy bar."

Again I pointed at it. "Whatchamacallit," I repeated.

"Phil," she said, getting a little agitated, "what's up with you? I told you no. Besides, you're a diabetic, you shouldn't even have it anyway."

I pointed a third time. "Whatcha . . ." My eyes rolled back in my head and I passed out on the floor.

I woke up a while later, surrounded by paramedics. Luckily, my mom's efforts every year to remind my school principals about my condition and what to do in the event of an emergency paid off. Jane and the Spanish teacher—and almost everyone else in that room or the school that knew me—knew I was a diabetic, and knew I needed glucose instantly (they also had the sense to call 911 and report that I was in a diabetic shock). What had happened was that I was hypoglycemic—my blood sugar had gotten dangerously low. When that happens, you go into what I call a "hypo hangover." You're sort of there, but you're not. I vaguely remember what happened that day, but not all of it.

What I do remember is that the next time I saw Jane, I looked at her reproachfully. "This would never have happened if you had given me that Whatchamacallit." I was kidding—it *still* would have happened anyway, because the candy would have taken too long for my system to process; I'd needed glucose right away. But Jane broke down crying, thinking that in refusing to give me her candy bar she had almost killed me. "No, Jane, I was just kidding!" I tried to apologize, but I think she swung her handbag at me, and deservedly. We remained friends. In fact, I think everyone in that

Spanish class came to like me and my diabetes. For the rest of that year, whenever anybody got hungry, they'd pass a note to me to that effect. I would then tell the teacher that my blood sugar was getting low. She'd let me go across the street to the convenience store at the gas station, and I'd pick up food for everyone in the class—and get mine for free. Hey, who said being a diabetic doesn't pay?

Back on the roads—which is what really mattered to me—the stage was set for a great climax to my first season as a serious racer. The plan was that we'd all go to Twilight, in Athens, Georgia, and I would qualify that afternoon for the prestigious night race under the lights. Then, we'd be off to far-off Cincinnati to compete in the national juniors' championships. The goal there: a top-ten finish.

A great plan, except for one problem: it completely fell apart.

All the improvements I'd made that winter, all the savvy I thought I'd acquired, all the lessons learned from Louis, all the fitness I'd developed—it all evaporated like sweat in two stunningly bad, anticlimactic weekends. At Twilight, you had to finish in the top ten in the preliminary race in order to qualify for the big show under the lights. I finished eleventh. I tried to shake that off for the national championships. I drove up with Louis, who was also competing. We both had high hopes, and we both got piss-poor results.

I didn't even finish, and that's about all I remember.

The summer before my senior year in high school, I finally, *finally* hit puberty. My voice got deeper, my muscles more defined, and, most important, I got a vehicle. It was a piece-of-crap car—a 1988 Chevy Blazer with about 110,000 miles on it—but it was *my* car. I had saved up all summer for it (working at Door Products again), bought it from a bike racer for thirty-five hundred dollars, a huge chunk of change for me in those days. For a lot of seventeen-year-olds, that car would have become their primary mode of transportation, preferably for the conveyance of young females. For me, the car meant that I could now drive to races. While I certainly would have liked to have women riding next to me, the first to get a ride, after my mom (who wanted to make sure, I think, that the car wouldn't fall apart in a block or two), were . . . yeah, you guessed it . . . a bunch of bike racers.

I had a new mentor now, along with Louis. Jason Snow was the real deal—a native of New Bedford, Massachusetts, he was a three-time national criterium champion in the early 1990s; he had also had great success on the roads and tracks. He had competed in Europe and had even won a race I'd heard of—the Tour of Somerville (New Jersey), the oldest bike race in America.

In 1996, Jason had been hit by a car while training and had to have brain surgery. When I heard that he had moved to Tallahassee and planned to race the Florida winter circuit as part of a comeback effort in 1999, I was thrilled. A pro like Jason Snow right here in my hometown! I figured that the guy they called Snowman could help push me up another notch in the cycling hierarchy. Under the assumption that my Publix experience had enabled me to make small talk with NFL players, rock stars, and grandmas—so why not a pro bike racer?—I brazenly introduced myself to him after a race. I remember being pretty cool and calm, offering him an outstretched hand and my signature "how are *you* today?" icebreaker.

Jason remembers it a bit differently. "I'd just won the field sprint," he says, "and this kid comes up to me all starry-eyed and says, 'You're my hero, man.' I was like . . . yeah, uh, okay, thanks, whatever."

However it went down that day, we were soon chatting and friendly. When Jason started showing up at the Food Lion rides in

Tally, I stuck to him like salt on a spoonful of grits. I think he soon picked up what everybody since Kevin Davis in racquetball had noticed about me: I was ready to do anything, go anywhere, and outwork anybody in order to achieve success in the sport. "Phil wasn't a really physically gifted person," Jason says, "so he had to use every trick out there to get to the finish line first."

It still smarts a bit to hear Jason's candid assessment of me, but he's right. However, I also know that the greatest champions in any sport are not always the most talented. I came to the conclusion that not only did I have to outwork everyone else, I needed to out-think them, as well.

Jason would show me how.

Soon we were driving to races together (occasionally in my car). The first time we drove together, to a race in Palatka, near Jacksonville, he said to me, "Okay, Phil, what are we doing today?"

I thought it was some kind of trick question. "Dunno," I replied. "Going to a race?"

He sighed. "No, Phil, I'm asking you what you're planning to do *at* the race . . . what's your strategy?"

"Dunno."

"Okay, well, I'll tell you. We're going to practice floating."

" 'Floating'?"

"Watch how I float in the race, and see how I position myself to save energy and use it later on when it really counts."

I watched Jason in the pro race that day and saw what he meant. In a race, riders tend to brake at turns, because they're following the wheel in front of them and don't want to lose that contact. But Jason would take a wide angle on these corners, riding (floating) outside the guys right in front of him, and then slot himself back in. He did this calmly, fluidly, and didn't begin his floating until near the end of the race, as I observed that day.

With five laps to go, Jason was dead last. *Boy, he's going to be pissed,* I thought, watching him from the sidelines. But on the next lap, he floated his way up ten places. "Wow," I said. On the next lap, he advanced another twenty places. With two laps to go, he was the fifteenth wheel. On the last lap, he was in the top ten. I started cheering. "Go, Snowman, go!" I yelled. I saw the pack come to the finish line, there was a field sprint—a gaggle of bikes and bodies rocking back and forth—and then the announcement over the PA: "Jason Snow is the winner." From last to first in five laps! Granted, this was an obscure winter competition in Florida, but I was jumping up and down, hollering like he'd just won an Olympic medal. It was more than the excitement of a great race that got me going—it was because I felt like *I* was in on the secret to his victory. Later, as were driving home, we talked about it.

"Phil, when you're racing, what are you constantly thinking about?"

"Besides Oreo Blizzards?"

"Seriously."

"Staying on the guy's wheel in front of me."

"Exactly. That's what most riders do. It becomes embedded in their heads. When you stop thinking that way, you can let a gap open and float back in and float back off. You don't have to constantly jam on your brakes and then accelerate again, so you're conserving energy."

It made sense. Soon I was floating around my competitors in the juniors' races when we turned corners, delighted with my success and taken with the idea that I now possessed some great bike-racing truth that the Snowman had revealed only to me.

One of Jason's other valuable lessons was on the easily said but harder-to-do principle of energy conservation. "Don't be stupid," he said. "Don't go blasting off at the start of the race, to show all the other riders what a stud you are. If you waste energy early on, you won't have it to use later." He taught me always to save something for the last five laps of a criterium. "By that time, everyone's legs hurt," he said. "But if you've been smart, you'll still have enough left in the tank to push at the end, when the other guys are on 'empty.' And that's how you'll win a race."

It's no surprise that today Jason is pro cycling director—the performance or racing coach—for the combined Mountain Khakis' Jittery Joe's team. I'm sure that a lot of the young pro cyclists in this generation are learning a great deal about racing from him. I was fortunate enough to have had him as my unofficial racing coach at a time when he was still racing. He was not signed at the time by one of the major pro teams, so he was long on wisdom and experience but pretty short on money. I knew that in Tally he was living with a buddy from Massachusetts on a temporary basis, so I invited him to stay at my mom's house. We had plenty of room and Joanna was always welcoming to my friends. She was with Jason, too, until she came face-to-face with the realities of the bike-racer world. In this world, at this level—as opposed to the relative handful of guys who have big sponsors or who race in Europe, where bicycling is a major sport—you're making just enough money to survive. Even when you're as good as Jason was. When you're not racing, you're training, and when you're not training, you're resting, in order to be ready to train and race.

Jason, as far as my mom was concerned, did an awful lot of resting. Maybe too much. "He's lying around here all day!" she would complain to me when she came home from work to find him with his feet up on the sofa, watching TV. I tried to explain that he had to conserve his energy for the last five laps of his next race, and besides, he was helping me getting better. She'd just grumble about people getting real jobs, and what kind of a career was this, and how I'd better learn about responsibility and not end up like this guy. I defended my friend, but I have to admit she did have a point. Much as I liked and respected Louis and Jason, I knew that I wouldn't want to have to rely on the generosity of friends to have a roof over my head. I'd seen my mom struggle; I'd felt the effects of living in a house where we were always one big bill away from bankruptcy. It was becoming clear to me that I was going to need a real career. Even if that career involved sales, which I was beginning to think it might, selling any big-ticket item would require a college education.

There was another factor. Part of me wanted to leave Tallahassee right after graduation and head to Europe to race. I was sure that with Jason and Louis's connections, I could catch on with somebody. But once I did that—once I was no longer in school—I could no longer be on my mom's health insurance. For most guys in their late teens and early twenties, that wouldn't have been an issue. Who needs health insurance when you're an eighteen-year-old aspiring professional athlete? But it was different for me. No health insurance, no diabetes supplies. No diabetes supplies, I'm dead. Much as I tried to ignore it as a bike racer, much as I'd managed to keep it in check, this was one time that my disease got in the way.

I applied to three colleges: Washington University, in St. Louis, was what kids today would call their "reach" school. I'm not even sure why I was reaching, except that one of the guys I knew from the racing circuit had gone there and said it was cool. Pretty lame reason for applying to a college, I know, but in the end it didn't matter, because I didn't get in.

My "safe school" was Florida State, which I could have ridden my bike to from our house. But with all due respect to FSU, which is a fine institution, I knew that the last place I wanted to be for four more years was Tallahassee. I needed to leave and reinvent myself somewhere else—not so far away that my mom would freak out, but far enough where I'd be in completely new surroundings, with new people, who didn't know me as Phil, the diabetic; Phil, who didn't reach puberty until he was practically eighteen; Phil, the guy who had no father; or Phil, the weirdo, who never went out and partied at night like a normal teenager, but went to bed early and disappeared with a bunch of old dudes every weekend to . . . *what?* Ride his bike?

Athens was the answer. Athens, five hours north of Tallahassee—not too close, not too far. Athens, home to the great bike race I already knew. Oh yeah, Athens, home to University of Georgia, to which I also applied.

While I waited to find out where I'd be going to college, I continued to race. I was eager for another season to soak up information from Jason Snow, but suddenly, in late 1999, he announced that he was retiring. Having never really recovered from his head injury, he quite sensibly decided that he'd had enough. At the time, however, I was really ticked off. Retiring, when he could still be of use to me? The nerve of this guy! This was me as a selfish little prick. If it didn't help me, it was a bad decision. I had no empathy, never took other people's needs into account.

Still, I had to soldier on. I raced through the winter, looking this time to the end of the season, to redeeming myself at Twilight and the national juniors' championships. A few weeks before the race, I got the word that I was accepted at the University of Georgia. Seemed to me a good omen. In April, I'd be racing in what would become my new hometown in September. Because this was also my last season as a junior (I'd turned eighteen in January), a whole group of family and friends accompanied me to Athens for the race. Even Jason, no longer racing, came along. Knowing that he was watching gave me some extra motivation, not that I should have needed any. If you're a junior racer in the South, Twilight is the biggest race of the year. There were about thirty-five guys in my race, including Keith Norris, a hotshot junior from Miami. Norris was a national champ—he'd won in Cincinnati, the same race I'd had to drop out of. These were some of the best young bike racers in the country. And this was the night to prove, finally, that I belonged with them. To do that, I knew I had "go Snow," meaning that I had to be as cool in my race as Jason Snow had been in the race the season before, where I had watched him methodically move from last to first. I knew he was in the crowd watching, along with my mom, my brother, Louis, Ray, and some other friends. I wanted to show the Snowman that I had learned his lessons well.

I sat in the middle of the pack, and then with five laps to go, I put my game face on and started floating. With four laps to go, I'd advanced closer to the front. With three to go, I got a little worried that I was boxed in, so I attacked, and with two to go, I found myself back in good position. When we came out of the last turn, I was the fourth wheel. Perfect! I had the momentum, and I knew that I was a good field sprinter, so I gave it full gas and picked off the two guys ahead of me. At this point there was just one rider ahead of me: Norris, the national champ, the guy who had waxed my ass all winter long at the criterium races in Tampa and Gainesville. But this was Athens; this was my town, now. I blew past him. Out of the corner of my eye, I saw Keith turn and register surprise at my presence. I know what he was thinking: *How the hell did Southerland get up here?*

With the victory at Twilight, I really felt that I was hitting my stride. A couple of weeks later, I skipped my high school prom to compete in the state championships. I raced smart and strong, and as I crossed the finish at the end of the field sprint—where, once again, I'd beaten Keith Norris—I threw my arms up in the air with joy. A woman official rushed up to me. "Southerland, you're in second place. Norris, you're the winner."

"What?" I asked, totally confused.

"It's against the rules to take your hands off the handlebars in a juniors' race," she said.

"There's a rule that you can't take your hands off the bars? I see it happening all the time."

"Well, it shouldn't be happening. It's against the rules in juniors' races."

"Why? What's the point of such a stupid rule?"

She looked offended, as if she had personally written and lobbied for that rule. "Why, it's because you don't have the skills necessary to control the bike without your hands, and we could have a crash at the finish line."

I was almost speechless. "Don't have the skills . . . what the . . ."

It didn't matter. She had marched off, having exercised her authoritarian power. Keith looked almost embarrassed. "Sorry, Phil," he said.

"Not your fault," I said. And then as the stupidity of what had happened hit me, I went crazy. "It's bullshit!" I yelled, and pounded my handlebars until my knuckles bled through my gloves.

Desperate, I sought out E. J. Rogut, the top official, who was as usual in the middle of a crowd of people. He, too, looked almost embarrassed when I approached him. Having seen what happened, he excused himself from those around him and pulled me aside. "Phil, I want to help you, but a rule's a rule," he said. "And if I override her, she's going to be angry. You put 'first place' on your résumé.

I know you won that race, and if anyone ever disputes it, you give 'em my phone number and I'll tell 'em what happened."

Mr. Rogut was a good man; and he made me feel a little better . . . but just a little. I felt as I had two years earlier, when another official in another place—Ocala, Florida—had ruled that I could not continue the twelve-hour bike race because of a faulty light. It wasn't fair then, and I still wasn't good at dealing with perceived injustices now, over two years later, especially when the one being treated unjustly was me. In a different time and under different circumstances, this easily provoked rage would probably have led me to organize a group to burn down the ROTC building, march on the Capitol or hurl stones at a line of riot police. But this was a bike race. What was I going to do? Organize a sit-in at the finish line?

I got my revenge the best way I thought I could: By going balls to the wall that afternoon. This was a pro race, but heck, I figured I'd been learning from a pro, so again, I tried to stay cool and calm, applied my Snowman tactics, floated around the field, and sure enough, I was right behind the lead pack of pros for the field sprint, and finished sixth—a very respectable showing for a junior. I also couldn't help notice that the winner threw his hands up at the finish line—and sure enough, the official who'd penalized me for doing the same thing was standing right there. "Hey, he threw up his arms! Why don't you disqualify him, too?" I asked her.

"He's a pro," she responded. "They have experience and know what they're doing."

"Wait a minute," I continued. "I just got sixth place in a pro race, so don't I qualify as having that knowledge?"

"Nice try, kid. But what's done is done, and I hope you learned your lesson."

I did—and the lesson had nothing to do with handlebars. It

had to do with acceptance and keeping my emotions in check. *From now on,* I said to myself, *we don't let the decisions of the officials get the best of us. We ride as hard as we can, as smart as we can, and we take the results, whatever they are. No more adolescent temper tantrums. Doesn't accomplish anything, anyway.*

There is strength in numbers, however, and that season I became part of my first team. Bike racing is a team sport as much as it is an individual endeavor. Being asked is also a mark of respect. When Tim Henry, a young rider from Roswell, outside Atlanta, asked me to join a team he was forming, I immediately said yes. I liked Tim, and I liked his dad, Bill, a supportive father who was always there at the races, always willing to do you a favor. The other two riders were Travis Hagner and Saul Raisin; again, good young riders that I had competed against, and respected. We called ourselves the Velo Rockets and wore yellow jerseys with our team name emblazoned on them. We even had some sponsorship: I got a free pair of racing glasses and a helmet. *Wow, this is the big time,* I remember thinking.

That spring and summer, I raced not just as a kid from Tallahassee but as a proud member of the Rockets. I now had three other guys working with me in these races, and it improved everything. I went back to the Jacksonville race where I'd won the first time. I had just upgraded to cat 2, so I was riding in a race with my team, which was pretty exciting. The first day, I got dropped. The next day, with help from my teammates, I won the juniors' race, impulsively throwing my hands up in celebration. Nobody said a thing about that. The Velo Rockets were also there for my big race in Athens.

At about that time I had an opportunity to go to Europe—not as a bike racer but as part of a senior trip for Leon High School. It would be a great opportunity to travel out of the country, and the organizers had raised money, so I wouldn't have to pay much. Much as I longed to see London and Paris, the decision was surprisingly easy. The way I saw it, either I could spend three weeks with a bunch of people from high school that I had never really associated with anyway, or I could race in the nationals with my three teammates and the other racers, of all ages, who had really been my peer group as an adolescent.

That was an easy choice. The Velo Rockets meant more to me than the Leon High class of 2000. High school was a stage of my life that I was glad to be done with. I now had a summer of freedom, to train and race, before starting college in September.

July 2000: the United States Cycling Federation (USCF) Junior National Championships in Trexlertown, Pennsylvania. My last summer before college, my last opportunity to race in the junior nationals. My goal was to finish in the top ten.

Everybody was there: my family, my teammates, my teammates' families. Just before the start, I checked my blood sugar: it was near 300 . . . high. "Jack," I said to my brother, "run to the car and get my insulin." He sprinted to the parking lot and back, handing me my syringe just as we were being called out to the start of the race. There I was at the start line, injecting myself. I noticed a few riders looking at me strangely, as if to say, *Wow . . . so brazenly?*

"It's not what you think, guys," I finally said. "I'm a diabetic."

The race began, and the tension was palatable. This was the junior nationals, and for a lot of the eighteen-year-old riders, this would be our last chance to make a statement in this race. At about ten miles in, there's a blur of motion in front of me. A crash! Maybe I should have hit my brakes, but the next thing I know I've slammed into a guy, and suddenly I'm pitching over the handlebars of my bike. I spilled onto the pavement, blood spewing out of my elbows, and then there was intense pain as a guy rode over my left calf. I got back on my bike, tried to chase the rest of the rapidly vanishing pack, but I was too far behind and in too much pain. I rode shakily into a feed zone and quit. I could barely walk, I had big cuts on both elbows, and there was a huge hematoma in my left calf.

I spent most of the rest of that day and night icing my calf and gobbling ibuprofen. I was still hobbling and in pain the next morning. The criterium was the next day—my last and best chance to win a championship—and I was determined to be there.

"Phil, you don't have to do this race," Joanna said.

"No, Mom," I replied. "I *have* to do it. I've been working towards this all year."

The race started, and for the first half lap I felt as if I were ripping muscle tissue with every pedal stroke. But then adrenaline or pigheadedness took over. I was in a bike race and there was no time or room for any more pain. Early on, I got sucked into an attack that accomplished nothing. *Stupid, stupid, stupid,* I chastised myself. Conservation and timing had to be the name of the game, especially given the condition I was in. I remembered Jason Snow's advice: "You only have so many matches you can light in one given race, so use them wisely."

Because of my injury, I probably hadn't had a full book to start with today. Now, I was down to one or two matches left, one or two times that I could make a sustained effort. But when? With three or four laps to go, I was still sitting way in the back. The pain had returned, I was hesitant to burn my last match, and time was running out. At that point, my teammate Saul Raisin took over. "Come on, Phil," he said. "Get on my wheel."

⸌ was not a criterium specialist—he would go on to become a ⸍d-class road racer before a crash ended his career prematurely— ⸍t he knew how much this meant to his Velo Rockets teammate. ⸍ gritted my teeth and followed, for two laps. That got me into the top twenty. I had two more laps to pass ten guys, in order to achieve my goal. I shut everything out for those two last laps. Matches? Hell, I was burning anything I could get my hands on, including, I would imagine, some brain tissue.

On the last turn, I saw a gap between the two guys ahead of me and the finish line. This was it: the decisive moment, the move I had to make if I was going to snatch a top-ten finish in a race I probably had no business even starting, given my injuries. But I reached down, digging all the way into the sandy soil of Munson Hills, where I'd ridden my mountain bike as a fifteen-year-old. I tapped in to the deep reservoir of my anger and pride, jangled every root and live wire I could find in my mind and psyche. This last push was for everyone who doubted me; this was for the officials who'd screwed me, for the guys in high school who mocked my lack of pubic hair, for Phil Sr., who seemed to have dropped out of my race long ago. This was also for the guys on my team, not just Saul and the other Velo Rockets but the extended team. This was for Kevin Davis and Dr. Nancy Wright, for the guys at Revolutions, for Louis and Snowman; above all, this was for little Philbert, the punk kid that I knew I was leaving behind that day. This was his last chance to shine, his last chance to burn. He was all out of matches now.

Pedaling like a madman, I surged into the gap ahead of the other riders and crossed the finish line in eighth place.

"Not bad for a guy who couldn't walk yesterday," I laughed, as I hobbled over to the arms of my friends and family. My mom cried as she hugged me, my brother hooted and hollered, my team-mates and friends patted me on the back and smacked me on the helmet.

The hugs were farewells, too. The next week, I left for college orientation.

7

Junior the Punk

There are times when the bubble that represents the bounds of human possibility must be pressed on, pushed out, and made to bulge. In other words, a person ought to step out to his borders every now and then and have a look around. It's good for the heart, the soul, and the mind. If a person can fight his way back from the fringes, the effort will make one stronger.

—HUMBLE CHRONICLER, *Athens Winter Bike League Web site*

It didn't take long for me to make my first mistake as a freshman at the University of Georgia.

That summer, a guy I knew casually from the racing scene, a recent graduate from the university, suggested that I request McWhorter Hall for my housing assignment. He seemed to think this would be the right place for me. So that's what I asked for, imagining a building full of pretty coeds. Turned out that McWhorter was the athletic dorm for guys. Also, it was located on the south side of campus, far from the center of any of the action.

I showed up the last week of August 2000 and found that my roommate was a twenty-six-year-old sophomore who wasn't even really into sports. He was, however, a huge devotee of a then-popular online role-playing game called EverQuest. This was a new, emerging world at the time, and one I had no interest in. So, although we enjoyed a cordial relationship that year, I knew right away that my roommate and I were not going to be heading out together to taste the great experience of college life. Like a lot of the gamers of that era, he was somewhat socially awkward—as was I.

The first night I was there, I was unpacking and decorating my side of the room. My clothes, my computer, a Lance Armstrong poster. A group of guys appeared at the door and invited me to a party. I immediately accepted. *So it begins!* I thought. *The college party life! Awesome!*

A few hours later, I showed up at the room where this party was being held. There were a bunch of guys standing around, talking in grave and somber tones to one another. *Hmmm,* I thought. *Guess they haven't gotten this party started yet.* I walked up to one of the fellows who'd invited me. "Hey, glad you could make it," he said.

"Thanks for the invite," I said. "So where's the beer?"

He looked taken aback. "We don't have beer at our parties. We have pizza and Kool-Aid."

"Well, all right," I said, forcing a grin. "That's better than the dining hall, I bet!"

He smiled thinly in return, as I wondered just what I'd gotten myself. No beer? At a college-dorm party in Georgia? Maybe these guys were beyond beer. Perhaps they were wine connoisseurs—or, more likely, serious druggies? One way to find out—and maybe lighten the mood, as well: I whipped the belt off my jeans and tied it around my arm, like a junkie would do. "So who wants to party?" I yelled out. With that, I pulled out a needle and gave myself five units of insulin.

Dead silence. Mouths agape all around me. Obviously, this was some kind of major faux pas, so I hurried to clarify. "Just kidding, guys," I said. "I'm diabetic!"

There was a murmur of disapproval and they turned their backs on me. My roommate, who had arrived a few minutes after me, had seen my stunt and quickly drew me aside. "Phil, this is the Bible-study group," he said. "They probably didn't think that imitating a heroin addict was funny."

Bible-study group? I rolled my eyes. Oh, brother. Later, I discovered that they were nice guys. But they were also, for the most part, devout Christian fundamentalists. Growing up in the South, you meet a lot of people with such convictions, and I'd learned that they are very often decent and well meaning and do a lot of good things. Still, they were far from the culture of liberalism and NPR and Joanna that I'd been brought up in; and besides, going to church and praising Jesus was not something I was about to do, especially at age eighteen.

Back then, I was far more interested in sinning, and as quickly as possible. Which obviously was not going to happen at McWhorter. So I fell back on my Publix experience, where thought and careful practice had helped me to break out of my shell as an adolescent. I decided that every time I went to the dining hall—about three-quarters of a mile from McWhorter—I'd introduce myself to the prettiest girls I saw. I came up with five questions that I'd ask—a kind of one-sided speed dating, although no one called it that then. I figured these were topics any freshman would like to discuss.

Hi, I'm Phil, what's your name?
Where you from?
What are you thinking about majoring in?

How's your roommate?
What do you like to do for fun?

I memorized the questions and started the process. There was some rejection, sure—but that very first night in the freshman dining hall, I met at least one or two kids who answered all five questions, and then asked me some in return. I also remembered a lesson I'd learned from Bill Henry, father of one of my teammates on the Velo Rockets. Bill sold commercial roofing, and I knew he must be good at it because he was a very persuasive fellow. At some of the bike races, when he'd driven us, I noticed how he always seemed to get what we needed, in part because he had such a deft touch with people. Once, after watching him in action, I asked him for some tips on how to be an effective salesperson. "Phil, rule one is know your customer," he said. "And always remember everybody's name. Calling a person by their name makes a world of difference."

I made it a point to remember the name of every Jason and Jennifer, every Andrew and Heather I met in that dining hall over the first weeks of the semester. If we had breakfast, if we shook hands, heck, if you'd answered just one or two of my five questions, I would try to remember your name, and greet you by that name the next time I saw you. I'm sure some people noticed me and thought I was weird. "Have you seen that guy from McWhorter going around asking people questions . . . ?" But that was fine, because for the most part, my charm offensive seemed to be working. I met a few very nice young ladies that week, and I suspect I could have gotten a girlfriend then and there. But I held back, remembering the advice that Ray McNamara, whom I viewed as a man of the world, had given me before I left Tally: "Whatever you do, don't get a girlfriend the first year." His logic was that if you did, you'd be locked into one person. "Then you can't branch out," he said. "Come on, you want to be a little Philbert the rest of your life?"

I got his point, and so was careful to avoid any serious relationships for a while.

Slowly but surely I began to make friends in the dorm and around campus. But, as was often the case in my life, I found my best and most lasting friends outside the confines of school.

During my first week at Georgia, I dropped into the local bike shop, a place with the cheery name of Sunshine Cycles. I introduced myself to the guy at the front desk, who recognized me from Twilight. Soon I was engaged in conversation with the staff and a couple of the customers about racers we knew, rides we'd done, our favorite bikes and gear. *Boy,* I thought as I walked out an hour later, *I didn't even need to prepare any opening lines for these guys.* I felt right at home. The guy at Sunshine had told me about some group rides in Athens, and that weekend I showed up for a training ride with some of the local riders. Their center of gravity was a six-foot-tall rider with a confident voice and a honey-sweet accent. You could tell he was a good rider just by looking at him—rangy and lean, and with the ease in the saddle of someone who knew had to handle his wheels. I noticed, also, that at the start of the ride—in front of Jittery Joe's coffee shop, located in the leafy Five Points section of Athens—he seemed to be making the rounds, exchanging a pleasantry here, a shared anecdote there. He left people laughing.

Who is this guy? I wondered. *The mayor of Athens?*

He might as well have been. David Crowe was an Athens native who had started bike racing the way you would think a true Athenian should. As a senior in high school, Crowe—who was thirty-seven when I met him—had attended the very first Twilight

Criterium. "I watched these guys flying around the center of town, people screaming their heads off," he told me. "Right then and there, I said, 'Holy smokes! I want to do that.'" He did—and went on to become a pro racer. He told me the story after I'd introduced myself and we were pedaling side by side through the countryside surrounding Athens. "I was never a prolific winner in the pro ranks," he told me as I listened attentively (in part because he was the first bike racer I'd ever met who actually used the word *prolific*). "But I can hold my own . . . and hey, there's one other thing I'm really proud of, Junior."

Already I had a new nickname. And when I asked him what he was really proud of, he said, "I'm one of the very few people out there with a pro license who is actually working full-time."

Immediately my thoughts flashed back to Louis LaMarche carefully counting the money he'd won at a winter race, to make sure we had enough for gas to get back to Tallahassee; to Jason Snow, with his legs outstretched on my mom's couch because he couldn't afford a place of his own. Or the time after another one of those races in Jacksonville or Gainesville or somethingville, when Jason actually passed around a hat to collect enough money for me to buy dinner, since I hadn't won anything that day. The hat got filled because everyone knew and respected Jason and felt sorry for me. But *damn!* I thought—I didn't want to end up a dirt-poor pro bike racer, having to mooch off friends, always staying in the cheapest motels, eating at the crappiest fast food joints. That's how all the pros I'd known existed. Hand to mouth.

This guy Crowe certainly wasn't living like that. He had a house in the upscale Five Points section of Athens, a nice wife, and a nice car; he also had a successful law practice, and despite his modest statements about "holding his own," he was still a terrific rider, as I soon found out. He raced smart, attacked hard. Crowe was the king of the breakaway. He could sense when it was going to take place. He'd get people working together—and not only in the peloton. Crowe, I saw, seemed to be the glue that held the Athens bike community together. "If you know Crowe," another rider told me, "you know everybody." That was true. By the second or third time I rode with him, he was introducing me to people left and right. One in particular, a fellow called Canada Dave, was one of his closest cronies. Called that because . . . well, he was Canadian, Dave Irving was a tough guy and a smart rider in his own right, one of the best mountain bikers in Georgia.

Riding with Canada Dave brought me back to my past, mountain biking my way through the sandy soil of Tallahassee with the Revolutions guys as a young teenager.

Riding with David Crowe gave me a glimpse of a future, one in which perhaps, despite my stature, despite my diabetes, I *could* be a professional racer—but without the borderline poverty that seemed to pervade the ranks of the regional pros, like some rank smell.

"Junior, guys like Lance are an anomaly," he told me, using another word I'd never heard out of a bike racer's mouth. "If you're a professional, chances are you're not going to make much money."

Still, while Crowe and Canada Dave were expanding my horizons, I felt that in some senses I had traveled to another state in an effort to reinvent myself and ended up the same kid, in the same old same social order I'd had in Tallahassee. I was again the youngest; now almost nineteen years old, but riding with guys in their thirties. Once again, I realized that, despite all those "hi my name is Phil" efforts to develop relationships among my peers, I had naturally gravitated to the older crowd. Was this some kind of ongoing search for the father figure or the older brother I'd never had? Maybe. Or maybe having diabetes had forced me to grow up faster. Either way, I had never really stopped to give it much thought, and besides, I was now too busy and having too much fun to plop myself down on some psychologist's couch to find out. A lot of the eighteen-year-olds I met—like eighteen-year-olds everywhere—seemed like idiots to me. Crowe and Canada Dave (like Ray and Jason) were smarter, cooler. There was much more to be learned from them. Under their mentorship, my education as a bike racer was proceeding well. I couldn't really say the same about my education in the classroom.

Like most freshmen at UGA, I took a bunch of required classes that first semester, and learned very quickly that if I read the textbooks, I'd fall asleep. So I tried to pay attention in class and take good notes. That was a challenge, particularly in Economics 101, which began at 8:00 A.M. The professor lectured in a monotone and droned on for an hour and a half about price elasticity, GDP, supply and demand. It was all I could do to stay awake. The philosophy class was better—the instructor was smoking hot, and I often found myself wondering how she'd look in one of those flimsy Greek tunics that they wore in the days of Socrates and Plato.

Truth is, I can't blame the faculty—or at least not all of them—or the subject matter. I did what I needed to do to get by; got Bs and Cs and was satisfied with that. I guess I figured that just passing and getting a degree would ensure the kind of career success Crowe enjoyed, overlooking the fact that he'd gone to law school. I gave little or no thought to where my classes were leading; a big mistake, as I would find out later. My training rides were far more important. That's where I was getting prepped for what I was told was the biggest thing in Athens since the B-52s: the Athens Winter Bike League.

"Junior, you need to try and win the WBL," Crowe said. "You do that, you'll come into the spring racing season red hot."

The WBL was like the Tour de France of Athens. Organized in 1997, it was ostensibly a series of four six-hour training rides from December to February, starting every Saturday morning at ten in front of Sunshine Cycles. But it was more than just a series of winter rides. The WBL had its own Web site, its own heroes (the Zealots), even its own chronicler. It was a wonderful bunch of eccentric, crazy bike racers of various ability levels, and I soon became part of them—and eventually, for reasons that will be explained, a WBL legend.

The first race of the winter series was in early December, and I was psyched. Still, the season opener was eighty miles. Despite all my training that autumn, I didn't have a lot of eighty-mile rides in my legs. Crowe and Canada Dave talked me through it. Although the courses varied, the structure of every race in the winter series was similar. For most of it, we'd ride hard but at a controlled pace. Then, about seven or eight miles from the finish, Crowe would blow a whistle. That was the signal that the attack zone was open. He did it in order to prevent a mass sprint finish on an open road (an invitation to disaster). Still, what it meant was that for nearly the last ten miles, the ride became a full-on race. Whoever was the fastest and smartest that day—a solo rider, a group, a couple of riders working together (or not!)—would cross the finish line first. That finish, by the way, was always at a different point along the Athens–Clarke County line. During that first ride in the 2000–2001 Winter Bike League, Canada Dave and another local pro, Rusty Miller, took me to the bottom of the last hill, three hundred yards from the county line, and I went full gas, sprinting for the line. But another guy was faster that day, and I was second across, in my first race in the WBL.

I thought I'd disappointed Crowe and Canada Dave. Far from it. When I went by the bike store that week, some of the guys chuckled when I came in. "Hey, it's Junior the Punk!" they laughed. "We read about you."

Huh?

They showed me a two-page fax that an anonymous contributor had sent around. It was about the first race of the 2000–2001 season and talked about how a newcomer to the WBL, someone named Junior the Punk, had kicked butt the previous weekend. It went on to say that even though this Junior wouldn't have known the Athens–Clarke County line if he fell over it . . . which he almost did . . . the kid raced his guts out and finished second in a heroic field sprint . . . and so on.

As I learned later, Crowe was the unnamed correspondent. Eventually, under the pen name The Humble Chronicler, he would start posting his stories about the Winter Bike League rides and riders on the Web site—where many of them are archived to this day. While he didn't use my real name, either, it wasn't hard for anyone to figure out the identify of Junior the Punk. Although I'd grown a couple inches that fall, to five feet eight inches, I was still the boyish-looking UGA freshman. Every weekend for the rest of that season, I'd hear it. "Hey, it's Junior the Punk . . . what's up, Junior?"

I guess it was better than being called a little Philbert.

I started racking up points in the series. So even though I couldn't quite beat the older pros yet, I finished high enough that, just a few weeks into the season, I was awarded a yellow jersey— my first! Now I was motivated to do well in this series, just as Crowe and Canada Dave had probably suspected I would be.

Three days before the next race, I called Dave. We had been doing a regular training ride on Wednesdays, but that day the weather looked nasty: thirty-three degrees, overcast, and with rain in the forecast. "So you want to do it?" I asked Dave. "Hell yes," he said. "I want to show you the course for Saturday." That's all I needed to hear. "I'll be at your place in ten minutes."

Off we go, and about an hour and a half into our three-hour ride, the clouds thicken and a cold, December rain pours down on us. I wasn't prepared for this; I had no rain jacket, thin gloves, nothing. We were miles and miles outside of Athens, deep in the Georgia countryside, so there was no place I could go to buy any (besides, I probably didn't have any money to buy anything; I was still scraping by). There was nothing to do but keep riding. I was soaked, my bike was soaked. I couldn't shift gears and could barely apply the brakes. My teeth were chattering, my face was blue, and I felt that if I stopped pedaling, my legs would freeze right then and there. It seemed like hours and hours before we finally got back to downtown Athens. Canada Dave peeled off and went home. "You're sure you're okay?" he asked before he left. I just nodded, but I was lying. I was in trouble. When I arrived back at McWhorter and got off my bike, I was shaking from head to toe. My hand was trembling so badly, I couldn't even get the key into the lock of our door. My roommate heard me, opened the door, and saw me standing there, about to keel over. "Good God!" he exclaimed. "What happened?"

I asked him to please take my helmet and gloves off for me. With his help, I stripped down and got into bed. He threw blankets on me, then immediately got on the Internet. "You have stage-two hypothermia," he announced a few minutes later. "Stage three, we have to take you to the hospital." Then he realized—not only was I hypothermic, I was diabetic. "What's your blood sugar?" he asked. I didn't have the dexterity to check, so he did it for me. It was 36 mg/dl, dangerously low. He rushed over to the little refrigerator we had in our room and fished out a carton of orange juice.

It took an hour before I was able to get up and take a shower, and when I did, I stood under the hot water for a full thirty minutes. *Another close call,* I thought. Without my roommate, I could easily have ended up as Junior the Posthumous Punk. But later that night, once I was feeling back to normal, I began to look at my near-death experience in another way. I'd survived. I was harder, tougher. No one else in that race coming up on Saturday would have gone though what I'd experienced that day.

Three days later, the weather was similar—overcast and rain predicted, but it was thirty-five degrees—two degrees warmer than it had been on our training ride. An hour into the race, Crowe turned to me. He'd heard what happened on Wednesday, and, much as he liked to have fun with Junior the Punk, he cared about me. "Phil," he said, for once using my real name, "you could turn around now and go home. You'll earn a few points in the series, and no one will think twice about it. Everyone knows you had a close call the other day."

I looked hard at him. "Crowe," I said, "we came out here to ride, so let's ride!"

I meant it. I was ready for anything. What had nearly killed me most definitely made me stronger that day. Sure enough, the rain came again, but this time I was better prepared, in terms of my gear, but more important, in my mind-set. Everyone else around me was shivering, but I focused on the two-degree temperature difference. *It's not as bad as the other day, it's not as bad as the other day,* I kept telling myself.

I ended up in third place, behind two pros, both of whom were ten years older than I.

The legend of Junior the Punk grew that day. I knew that Crowe would be telling the story to everybody.

• • •

By the beginning of my second semester, I was ready to get out of the dorms. Here again, Crowe came to my rescue. He and his wife, Gay, invited me to live in their pool house. It was perfect—like a freestanding studio apartment—and at $350, including cable and utilities, it was a real bargain. I accepted, and happily lived the next few years as the Crowes' next-door neighbor. Meanwhile, I had finally found an activity at college that I could excel in: bike racing.

Like many colleges, the University of Georgia had a club cycling team. There were maybe fifty guys on it, most of them strong recreational riders. Few had the race experience I did, and so although our teams and races were not typically as competitive as many I had competed in, it was still a lot of fun to be riding for the university and wearing a Bulldogs jersey. I was neither Junior nor Punk in this league, more like the big fish in a small pond.

Yet, the same time as I was riding *for* Georgia, I was trying to figure out how to stay *in* Georgia.

Money—the perennial worry for my family—was a problem again. I had taken out a big loan for my first year—eighteen thousand dollars. But my mom told me she couldn't afford to cosign for another loan. In order to stay on, I had to establish residency, so that I could get the more affordable in-state tuition. Although my mom couldn't afford to give money, Joanna was always ready to give time and energy. She wrote an impassioned letter to the president's office, explaining our situation, my diabetes, my bike racing, and so forth. David Crowe also wrote a letter on my behalf, saying that I did indeed have an Athens, Georgia residence, off campus. A guy who worked in the president's office, Matt Winston, responded. "Come in and talk to me," he said.

I prepared and rehearsed my presentation and went in to meet him. His office was located on the North Campus, where the administrative big shots were; a place few freshmen would venture, unless they'd been caught with their pants down somewhere. But I knew this guy could help me, so I marched into his office. "Thanks for seeing me, Mr. Winston," I said, and launched into my speech. "I love the University of Georgia," I told him. And while I might not be an honors student, I told him, I was working hard, representing the university in a sport, becoming a member of the Athens community, and, I concluded, "I plan to do good things someday for the world, and when I do, I plan to thank the University of Georgia."

That last part was unscripted. I don't know why I said it—or what I meant. The truth was, I didn't really care much about the rest of the world. My friends and family, sure. Humankind, I guess, in a general sense. But at that point in my life it was still all about me. Me, making money. Me, finding a career. Above all, me, becoming a better bike racer.

The turning point was coming soon, but I didn't know that. I just knew I wanted to stay in Georgia, stay with Crowe and my bike-riding buddies, and I was willing to say or do almost anything to achieve that goal.

At the end of the presentation, Mr. Winston smiled and nodded. "Thanks, Phil," he said. "You've obviously got some people here who care for you. We'll try and do what we can."

Although it took a little while, as these things always do, he was as good as his word. A few months later, I got a letter saying that I would now be paying in-state tuition—about ten thousand dollars a year cheaper than what I'd been paying as an out-of-state student.

I was saved.

Still, I was broke. I knew I had to get a job in order to make even my modest rent and tuition payments. Somehow, I decided that waiting tables would be a great job for me. I made a list of the twenty restaurants in town that I'd want to work for. I got rejected by fifteen of them, before the manager at On the Border—a Tex-Mex restaurant—hired me on the spot. It was August 2001. Now my nights were spent memorizing the specials (there was a brownie dessert with ice cream; not sure how Tex-Mex it was, but it sure was good), making culinary suggestions ("Oh, I think you'd love our beef burritos"), and trying to get patrons to spend as much money as possible ("How about another round of margaritas here?").

That fall, I focused on getting stronger on the bike. The way to do it, Crowe taught me, was with plenty of "pulling." Let me explain: if you're out in the front of a pack in a bike race, with the wind in your face, you're expending 30 percent more energy than the riders behind you. That's why you'll never see Lance or one of the other Tour de France stars leading a pack until nearly the very end of the race. They know it's just inefficient; instead, they let the lesser riders, the support riders, lead the way.

That's racing. But in training, if you want to get better, you voluntarily head to the front. Because riding for mile after mile in the teeth of a stiff wind will make you stronger. That's what Crowe had me do on our weekend training runs that season. I'd pull, pull, pull, getting hammered by the wind until I was ready to fall off my bike. Then he'd let me drop to the back for a while before taking the lead again. "Let the Punk pull!" became the cry that fall. By December, when the Winter Bike League was ready to roll, I could have ridden into the teeth of a typhoon. We put that strength to the test in one of the hardest rides in the WBL: the ride to Toccoa, a town nestled amid the mountains in the northeast tip of Georgia. The central feature here is Currahee Mountain, 1,735 feet high. During World War II, the mountain was the site of a training camp for the so-called Currahee Rangers, an elite parachute regiment of the 101st Airborne, whose exploits were documented in a

book and in the HBO miniseries *Band of Brothers,* which was air-
ing at about the same time we did this ride. There was a radio tower
on the top of Currahee that you could see for miles. As we saw it
looming in the distance, Crowe, riding beside me, leaned over.

"Hey, Junior, see that tower up on the top of Currahee?"

I gulped. "Yeah?"

"We're going to sprint to the top."

As Crowe recalls, "For the next five or six miles, as we rode toward the tower, Phil kept looking up at it. I thought he was going
to poop his pants."

When we just rode by, I breathed a sigh of relief—and then
gave Crowe a sharp look. "Very funny," I said. "Trying to scare the
new guy."

He was laughing. "Yeah, Junior, it always works. Everybody's
scared to death by Currahee."

While we didn't race to the peak, we did climb a total of 7,700
feet and ride 135 miles that day. I took my turns pulling at the
front, and felt good; the months of pull training had really helped.
In the last, decisive half of the ride, I attacked and shredded the
group. The strongest pro in the Southeast at the time, a guy named
Max Finkbiner, eventually caught and passed me. I attacked six
miles from the finish line. Max came with me; we worked together
with one mile to go, then he took off. There were other fast guys
behind him, I knew, who were going to try to pass me, as well. *I'm
not going to let 'em,* I said to myself as I kept up my tempo. I was
cramping like crazy. This wasn't even really a race, and yet I was
experiencing some of the worst pain I'd ever endured—as bad as
the junior nationals, as bad as the twelve-hour mountain-bike ride.
Still, I managed to hang on for second, and beat the rest of the field
by more than ten seconds.

It was a huge moral victory for me: I'd gotten to the point

where I could ride at the front and still be competitive at the finish in a WBL ride well over one hundred miles long and in the mountains.

That night, I had to work at the restaurant. I was bleary-eyed near the end of my six-hour shift, but still pleased because I had accomplished my goal: I'd gotten stronger.

When I went away to college, my mom's biggest and oft-stated fear was that I'd get completely drunk, my blood sugar would plummet, and I'd die in my sleep. It's true that alcohol does lower blood sugar, so young diabetics are often urged not to drink. Plenty of college students, diabetics or not, choose not to indulge, and that's fine. But for many if not most students, the "don't drink" advice is just unrealistic. I know from my experience as a freshman that there was no way I was going to let my diabetes stop me from being a college kid—and let's face it, drinking is typically a part of the college experience. I'm not saying that's a good thing, but it's the truth.

On the flip side, if you're an adolescent with type 1, you have to remember that no matter how drunk you are, diabetes is still there, it doesn't go away. I had still not forgotten the awful summer day in high school when I got drunk and ended up having to mow the lawn while watering the grass with my vomit. While I knew I wanted to party in college, I also knew I didn't want to end up sick or, well, *dead,* so I took a few precautions, preparing for a night out almost as if it were a bike race: I would eat a big meal before going out, check my blood sugar before I left, and keep checking it, even at the bar. I also made sure I ate something before I went to sleep (to balance out the blood sugar), and perhaps most important, before we started drinking, I always reminded my friends that I was diabetic and gave them some simple instructions on what to do.

It worked, particularly during one of the nights when I really got hammered. I'm not proud that I drank to excess, or that I woke up with a hangover, but that I woke up, period—and still had fun and didn't feel stigmatized—was because my friends knew what to do. We'd had a bunch of shots at a bar and I got sick. They helped me back to my dorm, threw me in bed, and decided to check my blood sugar. They told me later that they set the sharpness of my needle to the deepest level and jabbed my finger ten times before they got a reading, but they finally did: 156. They shook me awake. "Phil, your blood sugar is 156, what's that mean?" I regained my senses enough to say that it was fine. They asked me again to make sure that they and I had understood one another clearly, and left a note on my phone to have me call one of these guys first thing in the morning, which I did.

I was proud of my buddies, and glad that I'd taken the time to explain to them what needed to be done. Again, I'm not advocating excess alcohol consumption by anyone. I'm just saying—particularly to college-age students—that if you choose to, just do it right, which means taking a few precautionary steps and choosing to party with responsible friends.

As it turned out, though, despite a couple of boozy nights, I never did do as much of that college partying as I had imagined. With the kind of schedule I was keeping, who had time?

My days would start at seven fifteen so that I could grab breakfast and get to my classes, most of which started at eight. I registered for all early-morning classes, not because I liked them but because it enabled me to get home by late morning and onto the bike for an afternoon training ride. I'd get home in time to shower, change, and show up at my job at On the Border, where I'd generally work until eleven or eleven thirty. Weekends, the same, except that the rides—often races—would be in the morning, and I'd cram in some studying before work.

It was a productive routine, but grinding. And so when I got an unexpected invitation, in the spring of 2002, from a promoter in New York to race in Europe, I jumped at it. I would be racing as part of a team called People's Cycling—which sounds very uplifting and egalitarian but in retrospect was a polite way of saying we were a bunch of people who cycled for very little money. I was happy to hear that my old nemesis from the Florida juniors' races, Daniel Holt, was also on the team. When we were teenagers, I didn't much like Daniel. His dad owned a big bike shop in Bradenton, called Ringling Cycles, and he and his brother—also a stud racer—seemed to have every advantage that I lacked. He also appeared to me, at the time, to have a chip on his shoulder that was almost as big as mine. Well, now that we were both wise, mature twenty-year-olds, the situation had changed. Talking with him at some of the college races (Daniel was at Marion College in Indianapolis), I realized that he was intelligent, a good listener, and a stand-up guy.

The Collegiate National cycling championships were held in Burlington, Vermont, that May—just a few days before the Tour of Ireland. I decided to compete there with the Georgia team and meet up with Daniel, who would be racing for his school. Then he and I would fly over to Ireland together. Vermont was going to be nothing but mountains. To prepare for it—and Ireland, which I knew would also have some hard climbs—I decided to train on Brasstown Bald, a mountain even more imposing than Currahee. Located in the Blue Ridge Mountains, Brasstown is 4,784 feet high—the highest mountain in the state. So high that you can see Atlanta in the distance. So high that astronomers have lugged telescopes up to the top to get a clearer view of passing comets. So high that it would later serve as the King of the Mountains stage finish in the Tour of Georgia (Levi Leipheimer won that stage in 2007).

Training on Brasstown, I thought, would make me a cinch to win or place highly in the college nationals.

On a bike, Brasstown is a 2.5-mile climb. It takes about twenty minutes to complete, and for most of that time you're out of the saddle, standing up, grinding the pedals. Most riders don't do Brasstown more than once a year. I did three repeats up that thing in one afternoon, six days before the nationals. I figured if some training was good, more had to be better, right? Wrong. At the nationals, my legs felt like jelly. They were still fried from Brasstown, and I finished way back in the pack. It was frustrating, embarrassing—and a powerful lesson in the dangers of overtraining.

At the end of the race, Daniel Holt and I boarded a plane together bound for Dublin. It was my first time out of the country, and being a bit of a stress-ball anyway, I couldn't sleep. We arrived in Ireland on a typically rainy morning, and we're off on an eight-day, thirteen-hundred-kilometer stage race around the country. I'd be racing four days in a row—something new to me—and in pouring rain, something all too familiar.

The level of competition was really high: on the first day, in which I finished thirty-fourth (out of about two hundred), the winner was a guy who'd won a gold medal in the 2000 Olympics. This was heady stuff—Junior the Punk, Phil the diabetic, racing with Olympians. I had another strong stage the second day. This was going to be great, I thought.

On the third day, the roof caved in.

You may have heard the term *bonked*. It's cycle-speak for when a rider's store of glycogen—the fuel in the muscles that keeps us going—runs dry. Whoever you are, bonking is a miserable experience; kind of like being in a car that runs out of gas on the parkway, except that *you* are the car, and you're sputtering and wheezing, and in pain, and with each pedal stroke, feeling your muscles grind to an excruciating and irrevocable shutdown. For a diabetic or nondiabetic, it's awful. The difference is that when you're a diabetic and you bonk, the consequences are potentially fatal. Because when you're out of glycogen, your blood sugar plummets; a dangerous situation for a diabetic, who has no natural defense against hypoglycemia.

Oh, and one other thing about bonking: it often comes without warning. No engine light flashes. Just a sudden onset of pain and fatigue that gets worse and worse.

At the beginning of the third stage of the race in Ireland, I remember feeling good. It was seventy miles of green pastures and rain, and then, suddenly . . . I couldn't push my pedals. I had a complete and utter sense of emptiness that started in my legs and spread through my entire body. The group left me, and I have only the vague sense of finishing. I do remember that Daniel and I went back to our host home that afternoon—we stayed each night in the houses of local residents along the course—and told them that we, particularly I, needed food right away, preferably carbs, the main source for glycogen. Some hearty Irish cereal, the type we'd been eating for breakfast along the way, would be perfect, I said.

"Sorry, lads," said our hostess. "Cereal's for breakfast. I can give you soup."

I knew that soup was not what I needed. I tried to explain, cajole, beg this woman for cereal, but she would not be moved. Cereal was for breakfast, it was not now breakfast time.

Eventually, almost two hours after the race ended, I finally got some food. Then I collapsed into sleep. Apparently, I went into a seizure in the middle of the night. I remember very little, but I know that if it weren't for Daniel, I might not be alive today. Here's how he remembers it:

. . .

*There were four us in a room, and I remember waking up at 6:00
A.M.—the sun was already up—and Phil's standing over me. His eyes
were kind of glassy. I said, "Phil, what the hell are you doing? I'm trying to sleep." He didn't respond, he just stood there, looked at me weird,
and I rolled over and tried to get back to sleep. I heard him walking
back over to his bed and I'm thinking,* That's really odd. *I turned and
looked at him. He was back in his bed, lying on his stomach, but with
one leg extended straight in the air, moving it up and down. That's a
hard movement to do when you're awake, much less semiconscious. I
whispered, "Phil, are you okay?" He didn't respond. Everybody else
was still asleep. Now I was starting to get alarmed. I got out of bed,
walked over to him, and shook him. He rolled over and looked at me
with this dead, blank stare. It was pretty bizarre. He was looking right
through me, and making grunting noises.*

*The fact that he was diabetic was now running through my mind. I
remembered he'd bonked the day before and figured that this was somehow related. Phil had told me what to do in case something like this ever
happened, although he certainly didn't describe the leg twitching and
dead eyes. I realized this could be low blood sugar. So I grabbed a packet
of energy gel and squeezed some into his mouth. He sucked in some, but
some of it got all over his face. It was chocolate gel, smeared all over
him, and I remember thinking that if this wasn't so serious it would
have been funny. There was some fruit in the room, too, and I grabbed
a pear and put it up to this mouth. He was responsive enough now
to start nibbling on that, even though I'm not sure he knew what was
going on.*

*At that point, I picked up his big, boxy blood-sugar monitor (the
thing was about four times the size of what they use today). I knew
where it was because it was constantly beeping and annoyed the hell
out of me. I pricked his finger with the needle attached to it, as he had*

shown me, and looked at the meter. It came up as 16. I knew that was low, but not until later did I realize how low. When I've told this story since to groups of diabetics, they're amazed when they hear. They'll say, "Wow, sixteen? I've never been lower than thirty."

Sixteen is like . . . you could die.

Anyway, all it took was that gel, maybe another, and some fruit, and Phil was awake and responsive. He took it from there, and I think he poured himself a glass of orange juice or something. It's amazing that he didn't lose consciousness or have a full-blown seizure. And had it happened with everybody in a deep sleep, we would have never known. I guess in his half-conscious state, he'd gone over to my bed to get help. He certainly doesn't remember that part, and so we'll never know. But I do know, or I learned later because Phil told me, that I had probably saved his life.

A key part of being a diabetic is choosing trustworthy, reliable friends that you can depend on in a crisis. I chose wisely with Daniel.

Later that morning, I was well out of danger but still not feeling great. Nonetheless, we had a race to do. I wanted to be a pro racer and this was part of it: showing up to ride even when you didn't want to. Not surprisingly, I didn't race very well that day or the day after (it didn't help that it ended up raining most of those days). By stage six, I began to feel better. The final day of the Tour of Ireland, the sun finally broke through at the start. I was so psyched, I didn't put on my rain gear. We went over two mountain passes, and I was feeling good. Then the clouds gathered and it began to rain again. In the last hour of the race, the temperature dropped from about fifty-five to a bone-chilling thirty-seven degrees. I think I was hypothermic, I was shivering so. Yet, I managed to win a field sprint. And although it was far from the top-ten finish I'd envisioned— it was more like top fifty—part of me felt lucky to be alive.

People have asked me what the reaction of the rest of the riders was when they heard what happened the night I had a seizure. The answer: we never told anyone. I didn't go around advertising the fact that I was diabetic. At that stage of my life, my attitude was, *Who cares if I'm a diabetic? I'm here to race bikes, so let's race.* That's what we continued to do that summer, back in the States. When we returned from Ireland, Daniel, my old Velo Rockets teammate Saul Raisin, and two other guys, Brad Davis and Jeff Austin, piled into a GMC Yukon with seven bikes and headed off to the Midwest to compete in the Tour of Ohio.

The five of us were at about the lowest level of professional sports you could find. Yes, technically we were "pros." But, as I understand the word, professionals usually get paid for their services. The other guys still had some support from home, but I knew Joanna couldn't help me monetarily at this point. My tip money from On the Border paid my rent, but not much more. I was flat broke—and on the first day of the tour, flat on my back. I'm sitting in the top ten at the start of this race, going thirty miles around the town of Chillicothe, Ohio. I was on the wheel of some big guy. Suddenly he does a hard swerve to the right, and I'm face-to-face with . . . a giant bale of hay. Hay! *You've got to be kidding me,* I thought as I barreled into it and face planted.

I must have been out for a few seconds, because the next thing I know people were around me, saying "don't move, don't move." My neck and my ribs were in agony, and I was vaguely conscious of other guys lying around me in various stages of distress. Turned out I had caused a thirty-bike pileup. The bale of hay—one of the weirdest road obstacles I'd ever encountered—was later moved back, to give the riders more room on that turn. Too late for me, however. As the ambulance crew arrived and set up a stretcher, Saul came over.

"Phil, you all right?"

"Yeah. Come visit me in the hospital."

I lay on that stretcher in the emergency room for four hours. Not sure why, but it hurt like hell because of my ribs. Still, when they finally took X-rays, they were just bruised, not broken. My teammates came by later and took me back to our down-market hotel. The trip was off to a very bad start. The next day we assessed the damage. Besides my ribs, my rear wheel was shattered, my handlebars were broken, and my helmet had cracked into a million pieces. Yet, we decided to go on. I borrowed somebody's helmet, somebody else's spare wheel, and took what little money I had and bought a new handlebar. That afternoon, I basically rebuilt my bike in time for stage two, which started at night. On my jerry-rigged bike and in pain every time I took a deep breath, I got dropped by the peloton pretty early. The third day, I finished even farther back. Now I was getting demoralized. This was like the Tour of Ireland, except with better weather and even less money.

When you come to a bike race and can't race your bike the way you usually do, you get dispirited, depressed . . . even bored. That attitude spreads quickly through a team. Soon we were bickering, quarreling. Daniel got sick, and that hurt us more. We were only five days into a trip that was supposed to last a month. We were broke. We were feeling awful. We were disgusted.

But we decided to give it one more shot. We drove northeast, all the way up to Fitchburg, Massachusetts, where we'd heard there was a money race. In retrospect, it was pretty pathetic. We were now less than low-level pros: we might as well have been the bike-racing world's equivalent of a broken-down vaudeville act, second-rate circus performers in search of a not-so-big top. We were like Spinal Tap in the famous mockumenatry, a washed-up rock band in its last throes, playing second bill to a puppet show at a theme park.

The only difference was that we were supposedly at the beginning of our careers, not the twilight. I was twenty, and growing weary with the life of a roadie.

Arriving in Fitchburg, I began to perk up. My ribs felt better. We were warmly welcomed and given nice rooms to stay in by one of the local host families. The race was a circuit—basically a long criterium, in this case a five-mile loop. Off we go, rubbing elbows with many of the big American pro teams. I'm in fiftieth place, and all of a sudden, at a stretch of road where we opened up our speeds to thirty-five miles per hour, I see ahead of me a guy looking to his right, as the guy next to him falls. He knocks over a guy behind him, who knocks over a guy behind him. It was like a row of dominoes headed right at me. Before I could mouth the words *oh no, not again!* I get nailed by the rider in front of me, and I go flying off my bike. I'm lying on the pavement with three bikes on top of me. And I waited for those riders to get themselves and their bikes off me. I recognized one of them: he was a pretty big name in bike racing. "Excuse me," I said politely, befitting his status. "Can you please get your bike off me?"

He answered in a high, shrill screech. "Oh, I'm *huuurrrt.*"

This was a guy who would go on to win stages of the Tour of Georgia, and stages of major European races, and here he is, sounding like a toddler with a boo-boo. I knew he wasn't seriously injured—his fall had been cushioned by landing on *me.* I got really angry at this prima donna. I'm on bottom—literally and figuratively—and *he's* bawling. I mustered my strength, pushed the bikes off, then took his bike (a particularly expensive one, I noted), picked it up, and threw it into a ditch on the side of the road. He cried some more.

"What did you do that for?" he wailed. "Why did you throw my bike in the ditch?"

"Because it was on top of me, I asked you to get it off me, and you didn't. Instead, you're crying like a two-year-old, when I'm the one that's hurt!"

I got on a spare bike and continued for a few more miles. But I couldn't breathe, I could barely pedal, and I was so angry I had to stop. And when I pulled over to the side of the road, I swear that for a few minutes I thought I was not only dropping out of a race but out of the sport. I'd had it with bike racing, with crashes, with bonking, with busting my butt and pushing myself to the point where I was cross-eyed with pain and effort and yet still seeing little or no rewards. All my training, all my planning, all my listening and trying to learn and studying tactics—where was it leading me to? A hospital emergency room in Chillicothe, Ohio? The pavement on a highway in Fitchburg, Massachusetts? Another year of debt, cheap motels, and lousy food?

I'm surprised I didn't start wailing right there along with that big-baby professional.

Dan was still sick—as it turned out later, he'd had tonsillitis the whole time. Despite that, he tried to reassure me. "C'mon, Phil," he said. "Let's go home." I agreed. Using his money, we rented a car and split.

On the long drive back to Georgia, I was mad at the sport, mad at the world, and most of all mad at myself. I cursed everyone and everything up and down, as Daniel sat patiently and listened, letting me vent. Finally, he said to me, "Phil, just control what you can control, and let go of the rest." Daniel later admitted that he had taken a psychology class that semester, in which the bestselling book *Don't Sweat the Small Stuff* was part of the required reading. Still, while it might not have a blinding or original insight into human behavior, I listened. This, after all, was the guy who'd saved my life. He knew me, and he was right. I was tightly wound, stressed out. I was primed for a fall. Come to think of it, the priming was done. I *had* fallen. Twice in five days!

I thought about what Daniel had said. Maybe he was right. Maybe the answer wasn't walking away from the sport I loved, throwing away all my hard work. I needed to change. I needed to be more patient, to do the things I was doing, then let the rest fall into place. If I did that, maybe something really good—the big race performance, the lucrative pro contract, the breakthrough that would transform my life—would finally materialize.

Incredibly, it soon did, although hardly in the shape or form I had expected.

8

The Great Burrito Challenge

My original goal in getting control of my diabetes was that
I wanted to beat Phil Southerland in a bike race.

—JOE ELDRIDGE

After the series of bike disasters that summer, it was nice to know
that some people still had confidence in me. At Crowe's urging, I
trained for and entered the WBL, feeling better than I had in a
year on the bike. Riding on a beautiful Orbea Lobular bike that
Micah Morlock, manager of Georgia Cycle Sports, had given me, I
began racking up points and wins. But nothing is ever easy in this
sport. In February 2003, I had a bad ride, and crashed. I remember
someone telling me, "The WBL is over for you." The next day was
a 110-mile ride, with the apt name of Hard Labor Creek. I needed
help (again), so I called my former teammate Saul Raisin. The de-
bacle of that summer in Ohio was now in the past.

"Saul," I said, "I need you tomorrow."

"Phil," he replied, "we're going to get you this win."

It was a cold, overcast day in late February, one of the last of the
fourteen races in the series, and I remember that of all the people,
the guy who had the best chance to beat me that day was Crowe.
When he blew the whistle to open up the attack zone, *he* was the

one who attacked—and hard. But Saul covered his move, putting me in position to win. Saul was with me for the last few miles, at the end of which was a kilometer-long gradual climb. Bless his heart, though, he pulled back in the sprint, allowing me to win. I racked up a ton of points that day and was now in a position to win the series the following week.

It was a sweet feeling to know that I was about to be the champion of the WBL. This was grassroots bike racing at its best—a group of devoted riders, competing at a high level on these ridiculously hard courses week after week. While there was prize money involved, the majority of the riders competed for nothing but personal satisfaction, an opportunity to challenge themselves. Most of them could have been at home, lounging in their easy chairs or (okay, I admit it) studying. But they were out on chill Georgia mornings, humping up mountains fifty miles from home, racing for little more than the respect of their peers. I felt almost honored to ride with these people. The WBL had become my Giro d 'Italia, and to this day I'm as proud of the fact that I won it as I am of almost anything else on my bike racer's résumé.

But winning the 2002–2003 WBL came at a cost.

The same weekend as the series-clinching Hard Labor Creek ride, there was a race in Florida for the UGA team. I passed. It seemed a no-brainer. I had already racked up a number of wins for the team during my time there. Winning the Winter Bike League was a bigger deal, plus I stood to make $750 for doing so. I figured my teammates at Georgia either understood that or didn't care. Turned out, they *didn't* understand that and they *did* care.

Two months after I'd won the WBL, in April 2003, I attended a team meeting to choose the riders who would represent UGA in the upcoming National Collegiate Cycling Championships in California.

It seemed to me a foregone conclusion that I'd be one of them. After all, I was acknowledged as the top rider on the squad, I was the
team captain, and I'd stood on the podium a number of times
wearing the Georgia jersey. But when they read the names of those
on the team, I wasn't one of them. "Hey," I said, "aren't you forget-
ting somebody?"

Some of my teammates looked down, not wanting to make eye
contact. I think they were embarrassed. But there were a few, one
guy in particular, who had no problem telling me that, in essence,
this was a mutiny—and, from their point of view, with good reason. "You missed the race in Gainesville to ride in the WBL," said
this guy. "Obviously, you don't care that much about this team, Phil.
You just want to be a pro . . . you want to make money doing this.
We just want to ride."

Steam must have come out of my ears. This particular young
guy came from a wealthy family; for him, getting his hands on
$750 was probably as easy as a phone call home. I felt that he had
no idea what it was like to grow up as I had, where money was always a struggle. There was another issue, too—the Georgia team,
like most clubs on campus, was supposed to do some service or
volunteer work, which I hadn't. Again, not to make excuses, but
while they were involved in whatever fund-raising they were
doing—and I'm sure it was for a good cause—I was scrambling
and fund-raising for the one cause I knew: myself. Yes, I was selfish, but that wasn't the only reason. I was hanging on the edge of
keeping it together as it was, with work, school, and riding. I had
no cushion, time-wise, financially, or any other way.

Most of these kids, even the ones I liked, really didn't understand that. Looking back, I should have handled it differently. I
should have just said, "You don't want me there? Fine, good luck."

Instead, I told them they were crazy, making a big mistake, ruining their chances of winning—and, on top of that, reminded them that they were all a bunch of spoiled babies with silver spoons firmly placed in their mouths. I ranted and raved about how important I was to this team, what a leader I was, how hard I'd worked in races. It didn't matter. It was very clear that they all saw me as a selfish bastard who was out only for himself.

I guess they were right. While I genuinely did want to compete and win for Georgia, I had no hesitation in putting my own goals ahead of the team's. As far as I was concerned, the bigger goal for me—the goal that might get me noticed, might help me get sponsors—was winning the WBL.

But, clearly, not being chosen to represent my team in the nationals bothered me. Even more so, when I saw where it was being held. The race that year was contested in Berkeley, California, on a course that seemed made-to-order for me. The criterium was pancake flat, which meant it would be fast. A lot of the college riders, I knew, didn't have my speed. The road-race part of the championships, held over the following days, was on a course with shorter climbs, not unlike the hill profiles around Athens. An advantage to me.

In short, here I had been dreaming of winning the collegiate nationals for three years, now I had the best opportunity to do so, and I was being denied—not because of a crash or an injury, not because of finances or work commitments, but because my teammates didn't want me to.

It was killing me. A few days after that meeting, we were supposed to compete as a team at the Southeastern Cycling Conference Championships (SECC). The night before that race, I went back again to my teammates, including the instigators of the coup (which is how I saw it), to plead my case. This time, I practically begged them to let me compete in the nationals. I was sorry I hadn't done that race with them. I was sorry I hadn't done my share of the fund-raising work. "Please," I said, in one of those admissions of vulnerability that is so difficult for a young man to make. "This means the world to me."

No dice.

I was back to being infuriated. I told me them they could all shove it and marched out of the hotel room. That night, a younger teammate of mine, Brian Bibbens—one of the few who had supported me vocally—had to listen to me whine and bitch, as I sucked down a six-pack of Guinness.

The next day, I was fueled by stout and revenge. I wished that for one day I could have torn off my Georgia jersey and raced as a bandit. But, instead, I rode on anger, and lapped half the field. In the last lap, Daniel Holt (who had transferred from Marion to Florida State) attacked. Another guy and I followed him. I came out of the last turn in third place, but took the field sprint and won the race. The whole thing was a symbolically raised third finger at my Georgia teammates. *You think I'm not good enough for the nationals, eh? I showed you.*

That, I thought, put a nice period at the end of my feud with the team. The season was over for me, and at that point I didn't know if I'd even come back again the next year. That seemed a long way off, anyway.

After the race, I was sitting in front of my car, checking my blood sugar. Another rider—a big guy with brown hair—came ambling by. He said he raced for Auburn, but at six-foot-two and about 240 pounds, he looked like he should be playing linebacker for them. "Hey, you got diabetes?" he asked, as he saw me check-

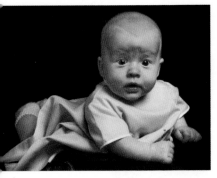

Knocking on death's door . . . lucky for me, he wasn't home.

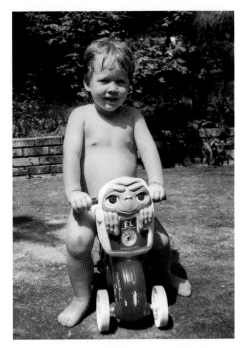

Not quite a Colnago, but damn it looks cool!

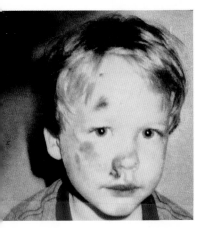

We all fall down, but getting back up is what defines you. The first of many crashes . . . learned early to protect the face.

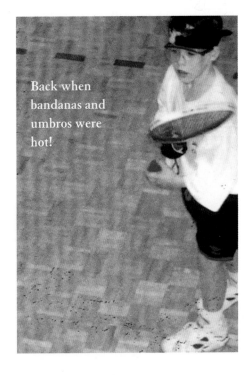

Back when bandanas and umbros were hot!

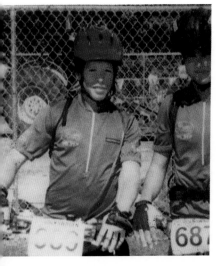

With my buddy, Jacob Mendelson, before one of my first races.

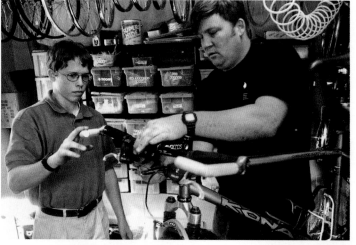

One of the rare occasions Ed Mill[e] was not throwing me in a trash can at one of my hangouts— Joe's Bike Shop.

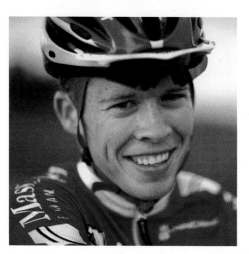

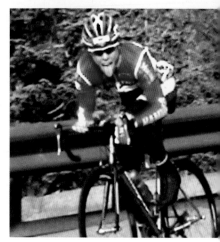

Left: I love my job! *Right:* My mom didn't like seeing me scream by at fifty-nine mp[h] down Wolf Creek Pass in Colorado.

The gun show begins. Shortly afterwards, Joe took control.

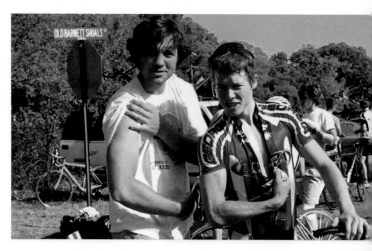

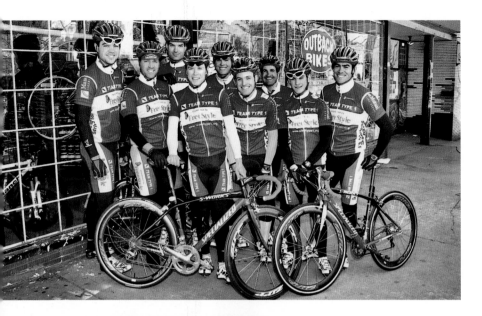

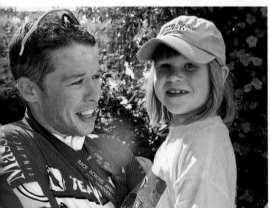

Top: The 2007 Championship Team at our first training camp in Atlanta, Georgia.

Center: I was so glad to have Heather see us finish RAAM.

Bottom: The first of many podiums for Team Type 1.

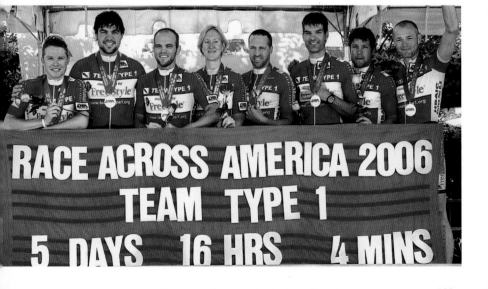

RACE ACROSS AMERICA 2006
TEAM TYPE 1
5 DAYS   16 HRS   4 MINS

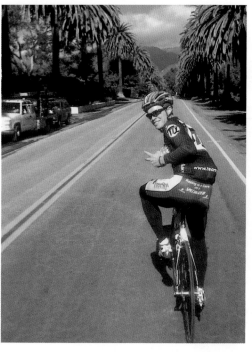

Paradise, Santa Barbara,
my favorite place in the world.

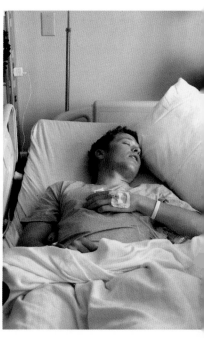

Post-op after my illiac endofibrosis
surgery, which was the beginning o
six weeks of hell.

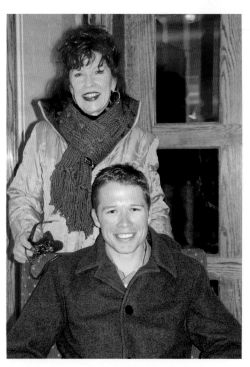

My creator and my hero, Joanna
Southerland. I love you, Mom!

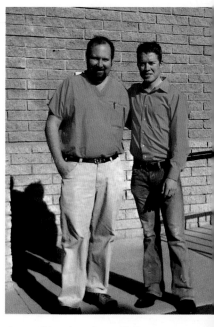

Great friend and top diabetes research
Howard Zisser, outside the Sansum Di
betes Research Institute—the first pla
insulin was delivered to in America.

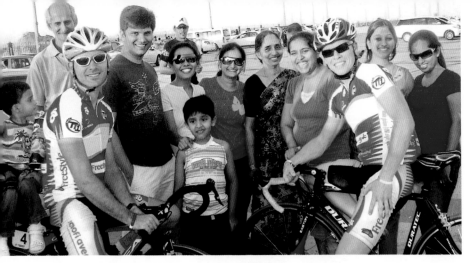

Our fan club after a seven-mile climb in the UAE.

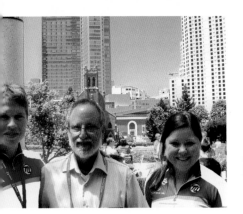

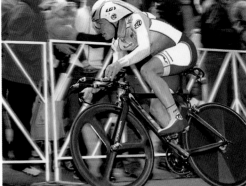

eft: My pediatric endocrinologist, Larry Deeb, and biggest success story and adopted
ster, Morgan Patton. I'm now working with Larry to get insulin to all children in the
orld. Right: Tour of California. If looks could kill, I still would have gotten crushed.

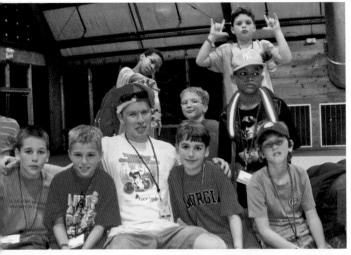

My favorite time of
year, every year—at
Camp Kudzu with
kids who all have
diabetes.

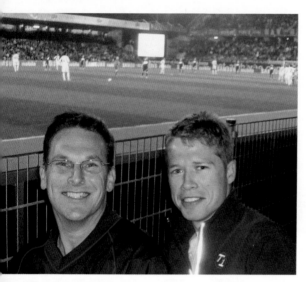

With top researcher for JDRF and fellow type 1, Aaron Kowalski, at a soccer game in Vienna. We make diabetes conferences fun!

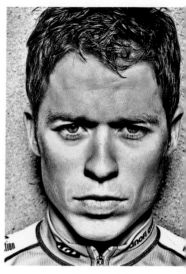

The 270th. "This is your last shot All photographers are the same even my good buddy John Segest

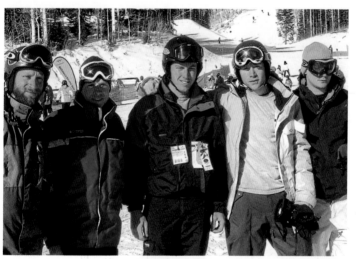

"The Wolf Pack" in Park City. Colby, Phil, Wes, Hank, and Matt.

With some of the best T1 athletes in the world: Joe, Martijn, and Javier in New York City.

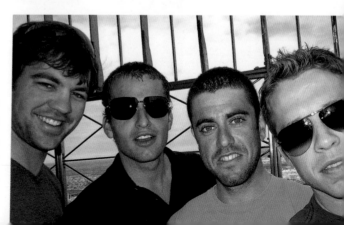

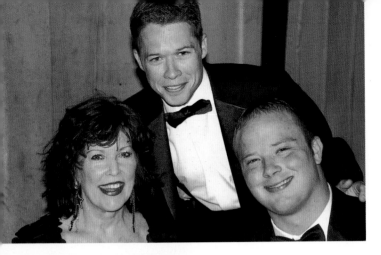

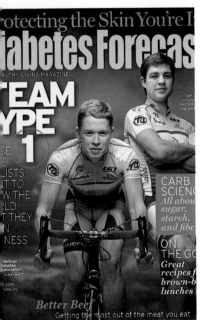

Top: With my mom and "little brother" Jack at the JDRF Gala, where I was a keynote speaker. Happy Mother's Day to my mom, as the gala was a day before Mother's Day.

Middle: We finally made it! The *Sports Illustrated* of diabetes! This was taken one month after I quit cycling. *Courtesy of Diabetes Forecast*

Bottom: Javier and me with the type 1 children of Morocco. This was another key turning point in my life.

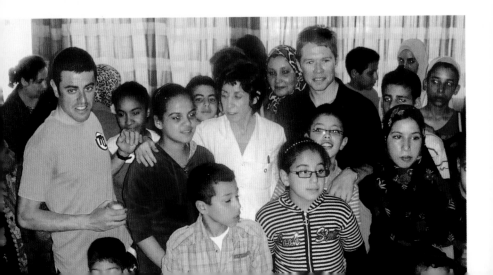

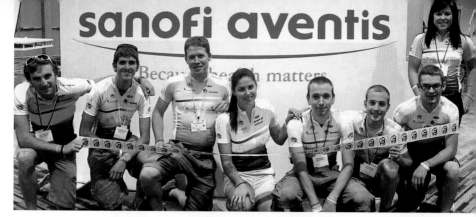

With the team at my favorite conference, Children with Diabetes, held in Orlando, Florida.

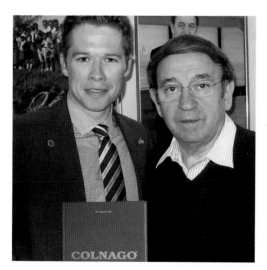

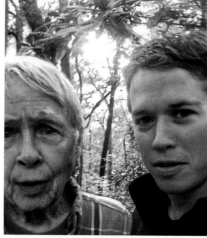

Left: With Ernesto Colnago, a true legend in the cycling world, just after signing o[...] contract extension. *Right:* The other half of me. With my dad, Philpott, Jr.

Below: With the President of Diabete Italia, Umberto, and the Sanofi team from Italy[...]

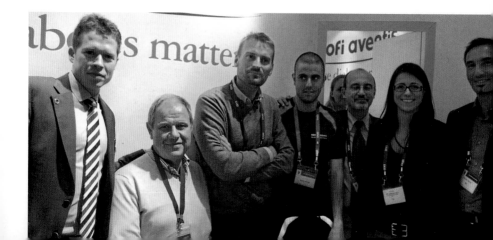

ing the readings. "No," I replied sarcastically. "Checking blood sugar is a hobby of mine." He looked slightly taken aback. I realized that I didn't have to be a wiseass to this guy. He had nothing to do with the Georgia cycling team. "Sorry, just kidding," I said. "Yeah, I'm diabetic."

He smiled. "Me too!" he said.

I'd never met another diabetic bike racer, nor had I really given it much thought. As usual, my disease was my concern, no one else's. It never really entered my mind to reach out to other type 1s, whether they were bike racers or not. "What was your blood sugar when you started the race today?" I asked, trying to make the diabetic bike racer's equivalent of small talk.

He shrugged. "I dunno."

"You don't know? How come?"

"I just . . . don't know. I don't really worry about it too much."

Another shocker: my diabetes, or, to be specific, the management of my diabetes, was always on my mind, if only to make sure that it wasn't hampering my performance on the bike. This guy seemed relaxed about it. Maybe too relaxed. Still, there was something about him I liked.

"Hey, I'm having lunch with a couple buddies. You want to join us?"

"Surrre," he drawled.

So the six-foot-two diabetic bicyclist-linebacker joined Junior the Punk, Daniel Holt, and a couple of other scrawny bike racers for lunch. We learned that his name was Joe Eldridge. He had grown up in Birmingham and spoke with an accent as rich and deep as the Alabama soil. He kind of reminded me of some of the guys back in the warehouse at Door Products—except this fellow was a college man and (so he would have us believe) a real hit with the ladies. He was also a lot of things I wasn't: relaxed and comfortable around people his own age (he didn't seem to need a list of ice-breaking questions to ask) and seemingly unperturbed by anything, least of all the fact that he had a potentially life-threatening disease.

Joe was ten years old when he was diagnosed with type 1 diabetes. In high school, he'd been diligent about checking his blood sugar and eating the right foods. Then he got to college, where it's easy to forget about such things. "I started making a lot of new friends, and they didn't know I had diabetes, so I never brought it up," he admitted later. "I guess I was kind of self-conscious about it."

Whatever the reasons, once your diabetes management starts to slip in college, it goes down faster than a keg of beer at a frat party. Joe didn't really want to talk about diabetes, anyway. Over lunch that day, he was more interested in telling us funny stories about growing up in the deep South. Alabama is as deep as it gets. To guys from smart college towns like Tallahassee or Athens, or from "Yankee Florida" cities like Bradenton, where Daniel grew up, Alabama is dumbed-down Dixie. The stereotype is that everyone from that state is a redneck, a cracker, or at best a defensive tackle. "Everybody thinks we're a bunch of country bumpkins and don't know how to do anything but hunt, fish, and play football," says Joe, recalling that day. "So I had to explain that some of those clichés aren't true . . . and some of them are even worse than they thought."

Although many of the stories are unprintable, Joe had us in stitches about guys he'd played high school football with, his coaches, his friends and their parents, and his neighbors. Despite all the *Hee Haw* humor, I sensed that Joe was a bright guy. His disarming good ol' boy personality wasn't quite an act, but he did know how to dial up the volume up on it, and seemed to charm everybody he met. At the end of the lunch, when he said he was going to be in Athens the following weekend for Twilight, I suggested we meet up and hang out.

The next weekend, Joe was there for the race—and so was his entire family, including his dad, who had an even better accent and told even funnier stories than his son. But he also told me something seriously: "You know, you're really an inspiration for Joe." Now it was my turn to be taken aback. "I am?" I said. At that point, I wasn't really thinking about inspiring anybody. I just wanted to ride faster.

Joe had just started riding a year earlier, so at that point he was not nearly the competitive racer he would later become. I was far more experienced. Indeed, he said that he knew me first not as a diabetic bike racer but as "that really fast guy from Georgia." So when it turned out that the guy from Georgia was also a diabetic— and one who was proactive about managing his disease—it made an impression. "I'd had a desire deep inside of me to change, and start taking better care of my diabetes," Joe says. "I needed someone to push me."

That weekend, a few of us went out to a bar in Athens. I noticed that before we got out of the car, Joe took a shot, and then left his diabetes stuff in the car. By contrast, I always had my meters, strips, and needles in the left pocket of my jeans—even in a bar. That way, I could monitor my blood sugar, depending on what I was eating or drinking, and adjust for it. Joe didn't care. Whatever his levels were when we got out of the car that evening, that's where he thought they were going to stay all night. At first, I figured that every diabetic has his own way of coping, so it was none of my business. But as the weeks went on, and we began to hang out more on weekends—and began riding together—I found myself growing more concerned about Joe's cavalier attitude. Joe needed a push, eh? Well, I was the guy for the job.

That alone was somewhat of a revelation. Me, care? About anything other than a field sprint or an opportunity for free bike gear; about somebody other than myself? Unusual. Yet, as we began to hang out frequently, I found myself lecturing Joe a bit about the importance of staying on top of his diabetes. I liked the guy, and I didn't want to see him get sick.

"Phil wore his diabetes on his sleeves," recalls Joe, speaking about those early days of our friendship. "He was busting out his meter, taking injections, and checking his blood sugar all the time, and not worried about where he was doing it. He didn't care if anybody saw him." Watching me, Joe says, "a little lightbulb went on in my head. But I quickly turned that lightbulb off."

I sensed that, too, and realized that just preaching about it wasn't going to change him. One night over dinner, I had an idea.

"All right, Joe, we're going to place some bets."

"On what, football?" he drawled, with a grin.

"No, on blood sugar. Whoever's got the higher blood sugar is paying for dinner."

"All right," he said, although I sensed some trepidation in his usually nonchalant voice.

We checked. Mine was 120, his was 200. "Fire up those burritos," I said triumphantly. "Because *you* are paying for dinner, my friend."

About an hour and a half later, after dinner, dessert, and a couple of drinks, I checked my blood sugar. Joe's nose crinkled. "What, again?'"

"Diabetes is different every day," I said. "You always have to double-check to make sure you do it right."

He shrugged, and followed suit. (I noticed that he had at least started bringing his blood sugar monitor along with him.) He was still around 200, while I had climbed to 150.

"Wow, I'm high," I said. "I gotta do another shot."

Joe looked surprised when I took out my insulin needle. "What are doing? Why are you taking another shot?"

I looked him in the eye. "I have a brother who doesn't have diabetes. Right now, his blood sugar is about ninety. If it takes me one shot or ten shots to get there . . . to ensure that I never go blind from diabetes . . . I will do it."

I saw the expression of shock on Joe's face. I could tell that he'd never really thought about it this way. Still, most changes unfold gradually, and so it did with Joe. We continued the betting system every week for the next three months, and I ate free for those three months. As we were both fans of Mexican food, that added up to a lot of burritos. But gradually the differences in our blood sugar levels began to level off. A couple of times I noticed that when I took a corrective shot, he did, too. He also mentioned to me that he had stopped snacking when his blood sugar was high. I realized that Joe had finally stopped denying his disease and had wheeled to face it. This was one of my first lessons in how change happens, especially for young diabetics.

Finally, one weekend in the early summer of 2004, Joe drove up from Auburn to visit me in Athens. We were now together pretty regularly, training, racing, going out and trying to meet girls. I was still living in the Crowes' pool house, and Joe came knocking on my door. I opened it and Joe barged in. "Hey, let's check," he said, without so much as a "how are you?" This was new! It was usually I who initiated the blood sugar comparison. We checked. Mine was about 110, and Joe's was in the 90s—the lowest I'd ever seen it.

For the first time, he had beaten me. He'd also cheated. The rule was that you didn't check until we met. But he'd done so four times on the drive from Atlanta to Athens and had even done a corrective shot an hour before he arrived at my door.

"I cheated to make sure I was going to be where I needed to win," Joe admits now. "Besides, I didn't have any money. I needed Phil to buy that night!"

I couldn't have cared less. I was so happy—and for once, the joy was not for me but for someone else. Off we went for dinner. For the first time, I picked up the check for the burritos. About an hour later, I look over and Joe is checking his blood sugar. He was around 150 (again, blood sugar spikes after a big meal, so this was normal).

"That's good, Joe," I said. "Especially for you, right after a meal."

He didn't say anything, but took out his insulin and gave himself a shot.

"What are you doing?" I said. "One fifty's not bad."

He looked me straight in the eye. "I have a brother, too, and he doesn't have diabetes, either. His blood sugar would be at ninety. That's where I need to be. If it takes one shot or ten to keep from going blind, that's what I'm going to do. You taught me that, Phil."

I was dumbfounded. Joe was speaking from the heart—not always an easy thing to do for a twenty-one-year-old former football player from Alabama.

"Because of you, I'm going to get to see my grandkids grow up." He thrust out his hand. "Thanks, Phil, you saved my life."

I think we shook hands, but I really can't remember—because at that moment, it seemed like a sack of bricks had hit me. My life changed.

• • •

I felt really good about what happened with Joe. And it wasn't the same good feeling I had after a ride or a race. This was a deep-seated satisfaction that I'd done something right, what my Jewish friends would call a "mitzvah." How right became even more evident over the next few weekends. I paid for a couple more dinners and realized that I couldn't afford these bets anymore. Joe's approach had totally changed. His diabetes management improved and, I began to notice, so did his cycling. This is something a lot of people don't realize: *controlling diabetes is hard, but once you figure it out, everything else in your life becomes easier. Everything else gets better.*

Suddenly, I had this need to connect with other diabetics and communicate the same message. I decided to try to reach out to people at the university, to see if I could make contact with other type 1 students and share with them the same things that had such an impact on Joe. I talked to someone at the UGA health center, and they put me in touch with a grad student named Meghan Moser. We met at a coffee shop in downtown Athens. She told me she was paying four hundred dollars a month for health insurance and another four hundred to five hundred dollars for her diabetes supplies and medication. For once, I was the person shocked by someone else's financial struggles. Because I was still on my mom's health plan, I didn't have to pay any premiums. But Meghan was a couple of years older and no longer eligible for her parent's plan—so she had to shell out eight hundred dollars a month on her own. A twenty-three-year-old grad student! That was astounding to me. (All the more so because I'd soon be in the same boat.)

Meghan and I also talked about control, the need for closer management. I emphasized to her that this wasn't about bike racing;

this was about taking better care of one's self, about paying attention and not ignoring the disease. While she was appreciative of the advice, I got the feeling that she was just happy to talk to someone who knew what it was like to have a disease whose presence imposed itself on you every day.

Speaking with Meghan and to other diabetics I began to meet over the next few weeks opened my eyes. First, I realized how many people with the disease really struggled. For me, it seemed that diabetes was almost easy. Life was the hard part. Socializing, controlling my anger, tempering my obsessive behavior, trying to succeed in my sport, and becoming financially secure—*that* was difficult. But type 1? Well, I'd just dealt with it—ever since the day long ago when my dad showed me how to inject myself and I accepted the condition as part of my life. That's not to say that I like being a diabetic, I just don't really have an alternative. Instead of being dominated by the disease, I'd learned to make it work for me, or at least not get in the way of doing what I wanted.

That wasn't the case for others. One girl I got connected with at the university couldn't figure it out and really didn't want to take the steps necessary to do so. She'd go to parties and wouldn't even bother to take her blood sugar meter or insulin. She had pretty crazy swings in her control. She also told me that the whole idea of her being diabetic seemed to upset her boyfriend, so she tried not to inject herself or even do a finger prick to check her blood sugar when she was around him. (*Would he be happier,* I thought as she told me this, *if she went into a coma or suffered kidney failure?*) I tried to give her advice similar to what I'd told Joe. She wasn't receptive to it. She asked questions, but I could tell that she was in denial about being diabetic.

That young lady was an exception. I found that a few of the other diabetic students I talked to seemed to admire me for the way

I'd refused to allow diabetes stand in the way of what I wanted to do. It seemed as if these young people had been waiting for a positive example, someone to look up to. I had been so wrapped up in getting better as a bike racer, so self-absorbed, that I never thought to connect or identify with any other diabetics. I now started to realize, however, that despite all my ups and downs in the sport, I had been fairly successful in the other, more important competition in my life: the ongoing effort to keep my diabetes under control. I recalled that at my last few checkups with Dr. Wright, my endocrinologist, she had praised my diabetes management; she had even used the words *role model*.

Role model. Me? Junior the Punk? Little Philbert? On one hand, I felt too awkward and inexperienced to be an example for anything except painful adolescence. Then again, maybe I'd been selling myself short. Maybe the part of my life that I *had* figured out—diabetes—could prove useful to others. Maybe this was my purpose in the world. Exactly what "this" was, I couldn't quite define yet—"diabetic role model" was not a job title I had ever heard of—but I felt that I was groping toward an important self-discovery, a new direction in my life.

My new helping attitude showed up in other ways. At the spring 2004 SECC Road Championships, I willingly played second fiddle to allow another teammate to win. His name was Todd Hendricksen. He was a freshman from Atlanta, a talented rider but a shy, somewhat sheltered kid. In some ways, I could relate to him, and now that I fancied myself a man of the world and an extrovert, I had made it my mission to help Todd—whom I genuinely liked—emerge from his shell. I took him out to a bar, tried to instruct him on what kind of opening lines to use with women, and I think I sparked what might have been the most scandalous, or perhaps exciting, moment of his life to that point. We were driving down to

Gainesville to one of our races, and on the interstate we saw a car full of attractive young ladies in the next lane. Todd shrank down in his seat, as I waved to the girls, mouthed the words *I love you* to one particularly fetching brunette, and then using hand gestures that I don't think I could or would ever try to reconstruct—especially while driving a car—I attempted to persuade her to remove her top. Amazingly, she obliged, flipping her shirt up and down and revealing her ample breasts for a split second. I could see her friends squealing with laughter. I also saw Todd's eyes bug out of his head. "That's how you do it!" I told him, trying to sound nonchalant, as if women were exposing themselves to me on a daily basis (truth was, I was as surprised as he was).

I hasten to add that this risqué incident was not the example of selflessness I was referring to with Todd. That came a few months later, in Athens, at the road championships.

Todd was racing really well at that point in the season, and I told him I'd support him. For once I was not "the man"—certainly not the prima donna who'd been essentially booted from the team the season before. Todd was a good rider, a good guy, and he deserved to win. I willingly became his supporting actor. I remember that last lap of the race there was a breakaway with six guys, including Todd and me. I knew this course well, and knew that there was a short, steep hill (a "popper," as we call it in bike racing), about one kilometer long, near the end. When we hit the hill, I let the four other guys do the work, while Todd stayed on my wheel. Then I attacked as hard as I could, to reel these guys in. They had been pooped by the popper—and that paved the way for my teammate to win. I took Todd to about two hundred yards from the finish line, then did the traditional "lead-out swing-off." This means that the guy in the lead, who's blocking the wind for someone behind him, swings off to give that rider a clear path to victory. I swung off and Todd went racing past me. I looked behind and saw that I had a gap between him and those four other guys. I dug as deep as I could, and finished second, behind Todd. It was a hell of a good feeling, because I'd done my job and helped a good guy win; but I'd also finished well.

I was changing. But before I could start to understand these changes, and where they were leading me, I needed a strong finish in another area of my life.

9

Thank You, Daniel Hopkins, Wherever You Are

I was beginning to see cancer as something I was given for the good of others.

—LANCE ARMSTRONG

In order for me to graduate at the end of the spring 2005 semester, I needed to pass a business finance class at the end of spring 2004. This was a hard class with a demanding professor, and I was hanging on the edge: I'd gotten a C on the first test, flunked the second, and received a D on the third. I had to do well on the fourth and final test in order to pass, and I had to pass in order to have a chance of graduating a year from then. I went to see the professor to get some extra help. He asked me my grades and I told him. He listened, and shook his head.

"No," he said flatly. "I'm not going to help you."

"Why not?"

"You performed so badly on those first three tests, you don't have a prayer of passing the fourth one. It's by far the hardest exam, so nothing I can do will help you at this point."

This absolutely lit a fire under my butt—which perhaps was his intent. I was determined to show this guy, just like I'd had to show every other person who doubted me. I studied like I had never done before. I read the chapters, did all the sample problems, read the chapters again, and did more sample problems. By the day of the test the following day, I had practically memorized the material and felt as prepared as I was for a big bike race. There were six hundred students in this lecture hall, taking the same test. When they gave me my copy of the exam and we were told to start, I attacked it like I would a course in the Winter Bike League. A couple of days, later, I got the results: 102. A perfect score. I couldn't resist taking my exam back to the professor's office. "Hi, remember me?" I asked. "I'm the guy you said would fail the test." I slapped the exam on his desk. "How about them apples?" I said. He looked at the grade, then looked up at me. "How did you do this?" he asked. "I just read the book," I responded. "I didn't do it with your help, that's for sure."

I marched out, feeling very proud of myself.

Now I needed a job, something that would pay but also give me experience in sales, which seemed to be the direction in which I was drifting. One morning, near my house, I noticed a sign for a company called LS Design. They did promotional T-shirts, business cards, and other so-called marketing materials for small and midsize companies. I dressed up, knocked on the door, walked in, and told them that I was the man they were looking for. The owner, Mark Czaplinski, hired me on a commission-only basis, and I made a sale early on, some T-shirts to some local business. That first sale gave me confidence that I could do this, that I could sell, and I ended up doing fairly well for them. I was able to pay my rent, pay for gas, and even have a little bit of money to take a pretty girl out to dinner. After a few months, he promoted me to vice president of marketing, so I was a student with a business card proclaiming me to be a vice president—albeit of a company of five.

Mark also didn't mind that his vice president made his sales calls on a motor scooter, which was what I was driving at that point. To save money, I'd bought a Japanese knock-off on eBay for $650. I got one hundred kilometers per gas tank, which held eight-tenths of a gallon of gas. I thought it was cool until a buddy wanted to take it for a spin. He put my bike helmet on and drove it around Athens, while I followed behind in his car. I was horrified at how dorky he looked on the scooter and worried that I probably appeared the same way. As it turned out, though, scooters got hot around Athens that year. You'd see these huge Georgia football players perched on these tiny scooters, putt-putting around town. As they looked far more ridiculous than I (although, of course, I would have never said so to the face of a six-foot-four, 300-pound lineman), I continued to make sales calls on my cheap scooter.

Still, there was still something making me uneasy about all this. Here I'd had this epiphany about wanting to help other people with diabetes, the way I had done with Joe, and yet I was busily preparing for a career as . . . what? An insurance salesman? A rep for some company? It just didn't sit well, particularly as I was now . . . finally . . . about to enter my last semester. It was December 2004. I'd be graduating the following May.

That was my state of mind as we wrapped up finals week for the fall semester. I'd been diligent with my studying, busy at my job, and there'd been precious little time for bike racing. Because I was restless, I needed to move, to think, to *ride*. A long ride. All the way . . . home? That was it! I called Joanna and said, "Mom, I'm riding my bike home for Christmas."

"You're crazy!" she said. "I'll pay to fly you down."

"It's fine, I'll ride," I said. "I need the training."

On the Wednesday before Christmas, I shipped a suitcase of

clothes down to Tallahassee. Two days later, I started out on my three-hundred-mile solo bike ride home.

Before I left, I swung by Canada Dave's place. He has this cool mapping software, and with it we planned out my ride. It was pretty simple, really—I took back roads, but there aren't all that many back roads in that part of Georgia, so the entire trip involved about fifteen turns. Dave and I figured it would take me two days: I could make 165 miles from Athens to the town of Montezuma, Georgia on the first night. I'd stay over there, then do the last 140 miles, to Tallahassee, the second day, arriving, if all went well, late in the afternoon of Saturday, December 18.

The night before leaving, I got my kit ready. Besides my bike clothes, I had Crowe's camelback—one of those water-filled bladders you wear on your back that allows you to sip through a straw while you ride—a change of underwear, my diabetes supplies, and a toothbrush.

With the directions taped to the stem of my bike, I pedaled out of Crowe's driveway at about eight thirty on Friday morning. It was cold, typical Winter Bike League weather, except that now I was riding alone into unknown territory on a ride I'd never done. When my feet went numb after just a few minutes, I began to think this wasn't such a hot idea. But my spirits climbed with the sun, and the farther south I went, the better I began to feel.

One of the beautiful things about exercise is how it sparks your creativity, helps you see things from fresh perspectives. As I rolled through the red-tinged countryside, ideas began flashing through my head. As a bike racer, Lance Armstrong was never too far out of the conversation, and I found myself thinking about Lance and what he'd done not only for American bike racing but, more important, for cancer patients everywhere. I'd read his book and, like so many others, been enormously inspired by how he'd beaten cancer. Diabetes didn't have anyone like that, I realized. No heroes, no big names that I could instantly think of and say, That's *my role model as a type 1 diabetic.* The closest one I could think of was Gary Hall, Jr., the gold-medal-winning Olympic swimmer who was diagnosed with type 1 diabetes when he was twenty-four. He was a great competitor—but his sport got noticed in the media only every four years.

Another concern, more practical but equally important, crossed my mind: health insurance. For diabetics, this has been a front-burner issue for years. We need health insurance to afford the insulin that keeps us alive. Yet, there was no group health insurance for diabetics.

I thought of Meghan, the grad student paying the eight hundred dollars per month for her health insurance. I also thought of the knock-down, drag-out battles I'd had with Joanna over this. There had been a couple of times when I had opportunities to race in Europe and possibly make some money. But she'd refused to let me go. If I was out of college for more than a semester, I was no longer eligible to be covered under her plan. It was for my own good, but of course I didn't want to hear that; I just saw an opportunity to race and get paid for it. In the end, she prevailed, and rightfully so. How sad, I thought as I pedaled down the country roads, that we should have even had that argument. No family should have to have that fight, and yet the families of diabetics in their late teens and early twenties must face this all the time—choosing between career opportunities or the need for continued health insurance.

Then again, the idea of "group" anything in the type 1 world rang hollow. As far as I could tell, there was really little sense of community among diabetics, period. I knew that was starting to change: the summer camps for kids by groups like the American

Diabetes Association were getting bigger and better organized. Still, as my experience attested to, one could live a very isolated life as a type 1 diabetic. Not necessarily a good thing. I started wondering how we could mobilize the diabetes community . . . create heroes and role models . . . unite all the 1.5 million people who battle type 1 and the 24 million with type 2?

I didn't have any specific answers as I pulled into a gas station to get some water and an energy bar. "Where are you riding to?" asked the clerk. I told him and his jaw dropped. "Montezuma? On a *bike*?" He and the other customers in the store couldn't believe that anyone could ride a bike that far.

At one point, after a long stretch of woods and empty road, I came to a crossroads. The sun was getting lower, and I did not want to be out after dark. But which way did I go? Somehow, this intersection hadn't shown up on Canada Dave's mapping software. I was also getting a bit foggy at this point. I'd covered 135 miles and still had about 30 more to go. Make the wrong turn here and I could be out riding in the dark, lost and in real trouble. I decided to make a right. It was a good guess. A couple of hours later, I arrived at the Budget Motel in Montezuma. I'd been riding for eight hours fifteen minutes and had covered 165 miles.

I still had no answers to the questions I'd raised in my mind about diabetes and what I could do, but I was beginning to connect some dots. I was now alert, amped up by the long ride, the productive explosion of thought, the feeling that I was groping toward something big. I called Joe and practically made a speech. "I have this idea that's been going through my head for hours. Something that you and I could do to help bring together the whole diabetes community. Let's unite people with diabetes! Let's get a group health-insurance plan! Let's use the bike as a platform, to help people take control, and get that group some health insurance."

There was a brief silence on the other end of the line.

"Sounds good." (I could always count on Joe for an expansive response. But I'd gotten to know him well enough to know that his mental wheels were turning, and that he would soon have some valuable insights to share.)

After that, I called my mom and told her I was alive and would be arriving in Tallahassee the next day, sometime before dark. Then, I went over to the Dairy Queen down the road, had an order of chicken fingers and french fries, and an Oreo Blizzard. *Okay,* I thought, *so maybe I won't be giving the nutrition talk if we put this team together.* The point was that I could eat like this and not have my blood sugar levels go haywire, because I was careful, managed it well, and trained like a nut.

The next morning, the soreness in my legs woke me up at six thirty. I changed, checked out of the motel, and rode my bike to a nearby McDonald's—the only thing open—in order to get as many calories in my body as possible for the day's ride. There was a gaggle of stout old gents in there, gathered around a table, sipping coffee. This looked to be their regular morning ritual. "Where you goin' on that bike, son?" one of them asked.

"Tallahassee, sir."

He almost choked on his java. "The hell you say," he sputtered. "You're riding a bike to Tallahassee? I get tired driving ma damn *car* to Tallahassee."

They all broke up laughing.

We chatted for a few more minutes, as I stuffed my face. They kept talking about how crazy it was; imagine, a guy riding a bike to Tallahassee! It made me think—riding a long distance impressed people. They would have looked blankly at me if I'd told them about my win in a criterium. They probably wouldn't even have known what that word meant. Attacks, field sprints, team tactics:

sure, the hard-core bike-racing fans liked that, and so did I, but the idea of riding vast distances on a bike is what seemed to catch the imagination of the average person. That was interesting and I made a mental note. I wanted to tell them that I was diabetic, as well, but figured that these guys could take only so much excitement in one morning.

We wished one another a merry Christmas and off I went. It was foggy and tricky to navigate. I had been riding for thirty minutes before I was sure I was going the right way. By then, the soreness in my legs had worn off and I was feeling good again. The temperature was in the high thirties, warmer than in Athens the day before, so I knew I was headed in the right direction: south. The flat land was as inviting as the climbing temperatures, and I went flying along at nineteen miles per hour. I zipped through small crossroads communities, past old plantations and cotton farms, along rows of pecan trees and long stretches of red clay fields.

Again, ideas spun through my head. Diabetes, health insurance, role models, inspiration, bike racing. I knew then that this could all somehow be connected—through some kind of organization or business—and that I was the guy to do it, with Joe's help.

The last hour of the day was the hardest, as I began to hit the rolling hills of northern Florida. By now my entire body was aching and I just wanted to get home. I rolled into my mom's driveway in Piedmont Park around 4:00 P.M. I was sunburned, my lips were blistered, and I was as hungry as a horse. Still, I was so excited about what had begun to crystallize in my mind that I had to tell my mom. We sat on the couch, as I sipped a recovery drink. I was two minutes into my pitch when she interrupted: "Where's your business plan?"

"A what?"

"You mean to tell me that after four and a half years of taking business classes at the University of Georgia, you don't know what a business plan is?"

I started to tell her about my busy work schedule and 8 A.M. economics classes, and she just waved her hand dismissively.

"A business plan is basic. And without one, you're going to fail. Oh," she added, "it would also be helpful to know what to call this new business or organization or whatever it is. Do you have a name?

I didn't, and called Joe. "Hey, Phil," he said, as soon as he heard my voice. "I've been thinking about what you said last night, and I think I've got a name for this organization: Team Type 1."

So, on December 18, 2004, Team Type 1 was formed. In our minds, at least.

The next morning, I joined some of my old Tally friends for a ride. All they could talk about was my three-hundred-mile solo trek from Athens. They asked me questions about the speed I'd maintained, the route I'd followed, how I'd stayed fueled up. I was impressed that they were so intrigued by the idea of an ultradistance bike ride, and yet, unlike the fellows at the McDonald's, they did know about bike racing. Something about the idea of an epic bike ride, across hundreds of miles, seemed to fire the imagination of all kinds of people.

Still, I was really jacked up over the idea of Team Type 1. Over the next few days, I told everybody about it.

My mom had a party at the house the night after I returned, and I blabbed about it to everybody. A Florida State professor listened and nodded.

"Good idea!" he said.

Neighbors and old friends listened and nodded.

"Wow, great idea, Phil," they said.

As I went on about it during our rides, the old Revolutions guys—my old Florida racing buddies—listened and nodded.

"Hey, what a cool idea," they said.

Only Ray McNamara told me what he was really thinking. "That's insane," he said. "Where the hell are you going to get the money to do this? Who's going to pay you to ride around the country and 'inspire' people?"

As was so often the case, Ray was telling me what I needed to hear. Just like everyone else, he genuinely wanted me to succeed (as he would prove soon enough, when he would play a key role in one of Team Type 1's early defining moments). But he didn't care about being polite or hurting my feelings.

Ray was right; Joanna was right, too. We needed more than good intentions, a vague idea, and a snappy name. We needed a plan, with specifics and details, and, above all, we needed money.

There was clearly work to do, and I was energized by the prospect of having finally found some direction in my life. The fact that I could ride my bike to get there was a bonus.

I took the bus back to Athens. It took me seventeen hours—about the same time it took me to ride my bike the same distance! Even a crummy Greyhound experience couldn't dampen my enthusiasm at this point, however. I was starting my last semester, I was ready to graduate, and finally I had a sense that I knew where I was going.

The first day of the semester, I sat down at a desk in a management class with Dr. James Epperson, professor of Agricultural and Applied Economics, who gave the overview of the course. "Just so you know," he said, as he went through the syllabus, "twenty-five percent of your grade will be the business plan that I'm going to ask you to write."

My ears perked up. I went to him right after class and started explaining my idea about an organization to help diabetics, and we'd call it Team Type 1 and it would involve bike racing, too, and . . . "Hold on," he said. "You have to pick something else, sorry. You're describing a not-for-profit organization. What we're looking for in the business plan is something that's sustainable and makes money."

I was crushed. This had seemed as if it was meant to happen. I pondered it and returned the next day for a second try. "Dr. Epperson," I said, "I'm going to start this organization and it's going to help a lot of people. So it's really important for me to use this for the class assignment." I went on to talk briefly about how the idea had been sparked when I'd helped Joe change the direction of his life, and how this, too, could be a life-saving organization, and explained to him the urgent need to develop group health-insurance plans for diabetics. I ended with "please."

He chuckled. "Okay, I'll make an exception," he said. "You can do your not-for-profit idea for your project." I thanked him, and before I turned to leave, he spoke again. "Let me tell you, son, you have the Midas touch."

Nothing that I'd touched at that point in my life had turned to gold, I thought. Maybe he was right—maybe that would change.

Part of the project for Dr. Epperson's class involved doing surveys—gathering market data to show that there was a need for your product or organization. I decided to do my surveys at the Mall of Georgia and figured I would piggyback it with a business trip I had to take there. While I was putting together the organization of Team Type 1, I still had pay to pay some bills. I had gone to a job fair on campus and met a fellow named William Brill—aka "Bub"—who had an insurance agency affiliated with MassMutual.

Bub and I hit it off, and he invited me to come up to interview for a position. No promises, but I figured that any interview at that point was good experience.

It was February 22, 2005, and my interview was at 11:00 A.M. I wore a Macy's suit that my mom had given me as a present for my twenty-third birthday, the month before. I borrowed a friend's car (my scooter wasn't up for this trip), left early for the hour-long drive from Athens to Atlanta, and arrived about forty-five minutes before my interview. This alone was a small miracle—in the Athens bike-racing culture, ten minutes late is early. On the other hand, I didn't want to be perceived as overly eager. I went into a Panera Bread shop by Bub's office and had a double espresso. I was brimming with confidence: I thought I looked sharp in my new suit and knew I could make a good impression. But a few minutes later, the doubts resurfaced: the idea of Team Type 1, of doing something with Joe and bike racing to help galvanize the diabetes community, just seemed an awful lot more exciting than selling life insurance, even for a successful guy like Bub and a big company like Mass-Mutual. I couldn't help feeling that way; it was almost as if I knew already that no matter what happened that morning, this was not my ultimate goal or my real calling.

I managed to banish those thoughts when I arrived at Bub's office. All cranked up on espresso, I rattled on about why I was uniquely qualified to sell insurance for MassMutual. Some of it was true. "I'm not afraid of the word *no,*" I said. "I have a good network of potential customers, I'm persistent, and I think I've learned how to be a good communicator." It seemed to go well. Bub said that this would be the first of four interviews. I knew it was going to be a bit of a process, getting approvals up the corporate hierarchy, but I had a good feeling.

I walked out of Bub's office feeling like a young man with a future. Now I had to change back into student mode. I'd brought my notebook and copies of my survey for Dr. Epperson's class. There was a Starbucks near the entrance to the Mall of Georgia, located about half the distance back to Athens. I'd scoped it out earlier and thought it would be an ideal place to conduct my market research. The assignment was that you had to interview ten people at random, explaining what your hypothetical business was and whether they would consider investing in it or, in my case, donating to it. It was a simple yes-or-no answer, and we had to just keep track of how many said what.

Getting anybody to respond either way wasn't easy. The first couple of people I approached just blew me off without even listening. They figured I was selling something. Some just shook their heads or said, "Sorry, I'm not interested," and kept walking. I didn't take that as "no" but as a "go away." Finally, a portly husband and wife stopped and listened gravely as I explained what I was doing. "We only give our money to Jesus," they explained. "And you should give all your money to him, too." They then asked me if I'd been saved.

That was it. I left the Mall of Georgia and drove across the road to another Starbucks. It was a good decision. The first guy I approached stopped and listened. "I have a niece with diabetes," he said. "I'd definitely support this."

I checked off the "yes" box on my form.

The next one listened and said, "Well, I give my money to cancer research."

That was a no.

Another couple of yes responses and then, of all people, I encountered a business professor from Michigan who happened to be on vacation, and who was naturally interested in my assignment and my organization. We had a really good conversation that ended with another yes checked off.

Finally, I went to this one guy who was sitting at a table just outside the entrance to the Starbucks. I remember he was smoking a cigarette as he sipped his coffee. He wore glasses, wasn't particularly well dressed, and looked as if he could have been a back-office guy on his break. I began my pitch and he listened, and then he abruptly turned it around. "If you had four hundred dollars right now, what would you do with it?" Huh? "Hypothetically, what would you do?"

I said, "Sir, I'm not asking for money. I'm doing this survey for a class to see if this organization I'd like to start someday is viable."

"I understand," he replied. "But just humor me. What would you do with four hundred dollars for your new business?"

I stammered for a few seconds, then replied, "Okay, I'd buy business cards, buy T-shirts to raise money and get the organization going."

"Good," he said. He reached into his pocket, produced his wallet, and took out four crisp hundred-dollar bills. "It's a great idea you've got there," he said, putting them into my hand. "Now go get started."

There was no big smile, no triumphant grin. Very businesslike. It seemed as if he had been sitting there waiting for me all along. I wasn't sure what to make of this. "Sir, I can't take your money," I said. He shook his head. "I'm going to put this money down here on the table," he said, which he did, securing the four bills under his empty coffee cup. "I'd highly recommend you take this and start your company . . . or someone else is going to have a very lucky morning at Starbucks."

"Okay, okay," I said. "I don't know how to thank you."

He waved his hand dismissively.

"Well, let's at least trade information," I said. "I'd like to keep you posted on our progress."

"Sure," he said with a grin. "Let's do that."

He wrote down my name and e-mail and phone number. And I took his. He said his name was Daniel Hopkins.

"Thanks again, Mr. Hopkins," I said, as he got up to leave. "This was so generous of you."

"Good luck, Phil," he said.

I left Starbucks and drove back to Athens. There, I went into the Bank of America branch in the Five Points. For the first time, I was asking about something other than what would happen if I bounced a check. "I want to open a business account," I told a teller. A banker, one Harry Binkow, came out from one of the offices and walked me through. He filled out some forms, got my EIN (essentially, a Social Security number for a business), and we opened a checking account. I told him about the team and what we were going to do, and he seemed genuinely interested. It was late afternoon by this time, but Harry stayed a half hour after closing time to finish up our business.

I walked out of there and looked at my watch. It was 4:30 P.M., February 22, 2005. Team Type 1 was now a reality.

From there I went directly to the office of LS Design. Mark, the owner, was still there. For once, I was the one who wanted to buy T-shirts. I explained to him what had happened and asked what he could do for me. "We'll sell 'em to you at cost," he said. "And business cards, too." After the fees of the bank, I had $387 from the $400 that Daniel Hopkins had given me. We ordered 100 T-shirts for $3 a pop and spent $56 on business cards. I had $31 left, but I knew that Daniel Hopkins expected his $400 to be used to help grow a business, not just left sitting in a checking account.

The next morning, I sent an e-mail to Mr. Hopkins, thanking him again and telling him that I'd opened an account for the business and ordered business cards and T-shirts. The message bounced back: undeliverable. I tried again, using several different combinations and spellings. Nothing. I called the phone number he'd given me. *"The number you have reached is not in service . . ."* This was odd. He'd mentioned something during our brief conversation about being in construction in Atlanta. I went on the Web and googled "Daniel Hopkins, Atlanta, Georgia." Still nothing. I tried "Daniel Hopkins, construction, Atlanta, Georgia." All kinds of variations on that. Still nothing. The man was a ghost. A chimera.

Later, when I told my mom, she told me the story about the physician, twenty-two years earlier, who had popped up out of nowhere in the hospital in Tampa and told her that while her infant son was fine, she was heading for a nervous breakdown. He'd further suggested that she would probably need to get a divorce if her husband was dealing with his son's diabetes by drinking. The advice changed her life. Despite repeated attempts to thank him, she was never able to reach the young physician, or even find anybody who knew a doctor who matched his description or remembered him being in the room that day.

Same thing with my mysterious benefactor. It was eerie. Still, whoever he is and wherever he is, I'll always be grateful to "Daniel Hopkins."

Over the next few weeks, I sold T-shirts for ten dollars to anyone who could breathe. They looked pretty cool, if I may say so. The designer at LS had come up with a nice Team Type 1 logo, with the slogan "Racing for a Cure" and our Web address. The Web site was designed by my mom (who, much to my surprise, had learned how to do this stuff at what I viewed as her advanced age. No offense, Mom!). It was basic but at that time served its purpose, which was simply to tell people who Joe and I were and—in the vaguest terms—what our mission was.

I started going to support groups around Athens and told people about our vague plans about changing the world for diabetics. There were few specifics. Still, I sensed that our enthusiasm was infectious. No one, least of all us, knew exactly where we were racing or what we were planning to do for diabetes, but by God, we were going to do *something*! Dave Eldridge, Joe's dad, gave us an idea on what that something could be: he had heard that the Juvenile Diabetes Research Foundation (JDRF) held a series of fundraising bike rides called the Ride to Cure and said that Joe and I ought to get in touch with the organizers to see if we could participate as members of the new Team Type 1.

Perfect.

The JDRF folks were thrilled to have us get involved. They invited us to come to Carmel, California, in May, to give a talk as well as be part of the ride.

As we boarded the plane for California, neither Joe nor Dave, nor myself or anyone associated with our nascent organization, realized that this was the first leg on the longest and most important ride of our lives.

10

The Race Across America

Every kind of weather, every kind of terrain, every kind
of logistical hassle, and every kind of body pain, plus the
lack of sleep, the ticking clock, paranoia, and widely
varying mood swings make this the ultimate cycling race.

—ULTRA CYCLING

Over the years, pundits, observers, and participants have exhausted
their vocabularies, taxed their store of clichés, and even bent the
rules of grammar trying to come up with words to describe the
Race Across America.

"Excess bordering on insanity."

"A breeding ground for champions, a testing ground for elite
riders, and a shining example of the strength of the human spirit."

"The most grueling endurance event in the world."

"Some call it crazy, some say it is unimaginable, and others
just look at you in disbelief and wonder why you would do such a
thing."

Well, I can respond to that last one. We did the Race Across
America not because we were gluttons for punishment, shining pil-
lars of humanity, or angling for sainthood in the church of endurance

sports. We did it because we could. And we wanted to demonstrate that to the world.

The 2006 Race Across America—or RAAM, as it's known—was everything it was cracked up to be: unimaginably hard, beyond sanity, the challenge of a lifetime.

But it put us on the map.

A big map, to be sure—one that stretched more than three thousand miles from Oceanside, California to Atlantic City, New Jersey. But at the end of that journey, we had arrived, in more ways than one.

That journey began a year earlier, in May 2005. I was talking to a group of about 180 children and adults that had assembled in Carmel, California for the Juvenile Diabetes Research Foundation's fund-raising Ride to Cure. The talk alone was a big deal. This was my first speech about Team Type 1. Barely six months had passed from the day that the idea had popped into my head, just three months from the day we'd deposited our first donation. For the first time, I was introduced as Phil Southerland, founder of Team Type 1.

I wrote the speech on the plane ride from Atlanta. I talked about our new team and what we hoped to accomplish—to show people what those of us with diabetes could achieve. Not surprisingly, it was a message that resonated with this audience, most of whom were diabetics themselves, or the parents or siblings of those who were. They cheered when I told them we would not let our diabetes stop us, because that's exactly how they felt. They wanted to know how they could join or support the team, and where they could see us ride. I didn't have too many ready answers for them at that point because, to be honest, Joe and I were still sort of putting this together as we went along.

The next morning, we went out on the one-hundred-mile, fund-raising bike ride. Cruising along the mountains into the Carmel Valley, I remember how spectacular the scenery was, and how hard the riding was, as well. A few generous donors—who also fancied themselves speedsters on the bike—heard that we were racing hotshots from back East. They picked up the pace and went scooting past us. Joe and I just continued to roll along steadily, and as the hills got harder, the breakaway artists began to drop, one by one, until it was just Joe and I. We didn't intend it as a statement about our abilities, but it ended up that way. Now, the people in the audience the night before would know we were the real deal. As far as what we could do to help raise awareness or change perceptions about the disease we all had in common, well, that was another story.

That night, the organizers put on a big dinner and party in the banquet hall at the local Best Western for everyone who had participated. Joe, myself, and a few of the ride leaders were sitting around, sipping beers and chatting. We were pumped by the way the talk had gone and pleased with our ride that day. There was a toast to Team Type 1. But we realized that clinking a few glasses and doing a couple of talks or fund-raising rides per year wasn't going to get us where we wanted to go. What would?

"You guys need to do something big," one of the riders suggested.

There were murmurs of agreement from around the table. "Yeah, big. Big."

Elise Rayner, a type 1 diabetic who was working for the JDRF, had been sitting quietly. Out of the blue, she looked up and said, "You know what you should do? You should ride your bikes across the country."

Joe and I laughed. "That's nuts," he said. "It would take forever."

Then something popped into mind. I had this fleeting image of a bicycling competition I'd read about. I looked at Joe and at Elise and said, "Forget about riding. Why don't we *race* across America?"

We all put down our drinks. We were onto something.

"If we could put a team of people with diabetes together and do the Race Across America, that would blow people away," I said. "Who would imagine that a bunch of diabetics could ever achieve something that difficult?"

"That would be awesome," Joe said.

"I love it," echoed Elise.

Not content to stop there, I raised the ante again: "We wouldn't just do this Race Across America," I said. "We'd have to *win* it."

Silence. If we had drawn thought balloons over Joe's and Elise's heads at the moment, what they were probably thinking was, *Great idea, Phil. But it'll never happen.*

They had every reason to be skeptical. What I was proposing was pure audacity on a number of levels. First, we didn't have a team—it was just Joe and I. Second, RAAM is a specialized event. Not Lance Armstrong, not Greg LeMond, not any of the great Tour de France riders had ever done it. Even for them—guys who routinely ride one hundred miles a day, up and down mountains— this was considered extreme, almost ludicrous, the province of a very specific class of athlete. These were the ultrariders, often solo, often . . . well, kind of weird and eccentric. The winners of RAAM tended to be iconoclasts. Eastern Europeans with hard faces and harder-to-pronounce names. Guys from the wilds of Alaska with beards. Cyclists who had done things like riding solo across Australia. Adventurers who had climbed Mount. Everest and were now looking for their next challenge.

Here we were, a couple of All-American-looking, bike-racing kids. Could we really compete with those grizzled endurance animals?

The answer was no—nor did we really want to. We were Team Type 1, accent on the "Team," and if we were going to do this race, we were going to do it as a team. Fortunately, RAAM could accommodate that. This is a pursuit with a long history of attracting crazies and dreamers.

Cross-country cycling began during the bicycle mania that swept America in the late nineteenth century. According to records kept by the Ultra Marathon Cycling Association, the first man to bike across the United States was an Englishman named Thomas Stevens, who rode one of those old-fashioned "penny farthing" bicycles from Oakland, California to Boston in the summer of 1884. It took him 104 days and six hours—some three and a half months! Three years later, a newspaperman, George Nellis, cut that time down dramatically. He traversed the United States on a forty-five-pound iron high-wheel bicycle with no gears and with pedals attached directly to the front wheel. Nellis, who followed the railroad routes that were then newly built, also made the crossing west to east, finishing in Boston in only eighty days.

A handful of individuals made the transcontinental bike trek over the ensuing decades, but they were eventually left in the exhaust fumes of Jack Kerouac and Neil Cassady's sleek Hudson, the sports cars of Route 66, Ken Kesey's school bus, and CB-squawking truckers balling all night across America's superhighways—all the iconic symbols of America's twentieth-century automotive culture (and being from the South, where that culture was famously celebrated and practiced, I do understand this). The notion of two-wheeled, nonmotorized cross-country travel seemed archaic, vaguely absurd. Why ride a bike when you could floor a Corvette?

It wasn't just ultracycling but competitive cycling that almost disappeared. In 1972, British writer Frederick Alderson lamented the decline of the sport in the United States. "The general preference by Americans for sports enjoyable in shorter bursts has left only two professional riders in the USA," he wrote in his book, *Bicycling: A History*.

That was about to change, and not because Americans were suddenly becoming more enamored of the great sport of bicycling racing per se. In the mid-1970s, amid rising interest in physical fitness, a guy named John Marino decided he needed a new challenge. Marino had been a star baseball and football player at Hollywood High School in California. His hometown team, the Los Angeles Dodgers, had drafted him, but he decided to go to San Diego State to pursue a teaching degree first. While there, he injured his back while weight training, putting an end to his baseball career. In 1976, Marino, restless and still ambitious, began paging through the *Guinness Book of World Records*. "I wanted to be in this book someday," he later told an interviewer. "I chose cycling and specifically the U.S. coast-to-coast record."

So the baller became a biker, a self-described "cycling fanatic," for two years, as he trained and prepared for his record-setting ride. He soon realized that there was more involved than his own endurance. Planning a ride across the country was more like an expedition than a competition. Food, equipment, support crew, extra bikes, weather, clothing, scheduling, sleep, routing, driving, vehicles—all of these factors had to be considered. By 1978, Marino was ready. He made the ride, from Santa Monica's City Hall to City Hall in lower Manhattan, and entered the record book, finishing in thirteen days, one hour, twenty minutes.

"Finishing that ride was the greatest thrill of my life," he recalled later, in an interview with the Web site ultracycling.com. "I had taken on a task that I hadn't a clue what to expect."

Marino realized that what he had done was also, in his own words, pretty "out there." But he sensed correctly that there were others out there who wanted to do something similarly challenging, spectacular, extreme. Along with contemporaries such as Fred Lebow, the visionary founder of the New York City Marathon, and John Collins, the retired navy captain credited with the idea of the Ironman Triathlon, Marino realized that in postwar, postsixties America, "if you created a sporting event believed to be the toughest and most grueling, people will stand in line to enter and pay you to do it."

He would be proved right.

In 1982, Marino raced across the United States again. This time, his competition wasn't the clock; it was three other ultracyclists— Lon Haldeman, Michael Shermer, and John Howard—who joined him in what was billed as the first "Great American Bike Race." ABC Sports got wind of it and contacted Marino. The network wanted to cover the race for their popular *Wide World of Sports* program. As the competition unfolded, and the five riders began to spread apart, Marino began to have second thoughts. "The race didn't involve any neck-and-neck drama," he recalled. "I thought that the whole thing was a mistake for ABC." He called the producers during one of his rest stops. To his surprise, he found that they were anything but disappointed. They weren't interested in the competition as much as the drama of five individuals taking on the breadth of the continent. That was the real story: men against the deserts, mountains, and plains of America—from one end to the other. While Haldeman was the winner that year, what was more important about the first race across America was that it was subsequently watched by much of America, in what became an award-winning segment of *Wide World of Sports.*

After a couple of years of broadcasting the event, which soon became known by the name that best described it—the Race Across America—ABC moved on to other offbeat sports. But that initial nationwide coverage gave RAAM the cachet it needed, believes Marino, who himself stayed with the race until 1992, the same year that *Outside* magazine ranked RAAM as the world's single toughest endurance event—ahead of such competitions as the Iditarod in Alaska, the Ironman Triathlon in Hawaii, and the Badwater Ultramarathon in Death Valley. That helped add to the event's mystique, and a new wave of adventurers and masochists began flocking to the race that had carved a niche for itself in the pantheon of endurance sports.

Over the years, the event expanded to include two-, four-, and eight-person teams. More women began to compete, and there were even categories added for riders on tandem and recumbent bikes. Still, while the field generally only numbers about 125 riders, it attracts thousands of spectators and considerable media interest along the way. With good reason. As Marino told ultracycling. com, RAAM's real appeal was "not the quantity of the entrants or the cyclists, it was the quality of the endeavor."

Now we were going to be part of it. As soon as I got back home to Atlanta from California, I began telling everybody that we were doing RAAM. That's how I tend to operate. Once I have an idea, I talk it up to everyone with an ear, and hope that by spreading the word through my network, I'll come up with the necessary resources. For starters, I posted e-mails on every diabetes Web site I could find, like this one, on diabetesmonitor.com:

*Hello, I would like to invite you to come watch Team Type 1 in
our Race Across America. Team Type 1 is comprised of eight
Type 1 diabetics, and we have the goal of breaking the record in
the Race. We also have the goal of raising $1,000,000 for the
Juvenile Diabetes Research Foundation this June. We would
love to have your support. Please visit www.teamtype1.org to
donate. We have new cool wristbands available, as well as an
online donation page. Thank you so much for your support.
Without you, this would not be possible.*

Pretty blunt, pretty forward . . . basically a "hi, give us money"
message. But again, we realized that we were preparing for something more than a bike race; this would be the event that would
help legitimize us. To do it successfully, we were going to need every penny and every ounce of support we could get.

First, I had another priority, however: a week as a counselor at
Camp Kudzu. Founded by a group of parents, health professionals, and community leaders, Kudzu was a summer camp for kids
with type 1. Since its inception six years earlier, in 1999, the number of campers, programs, and volunteers had continued, as the
organizers like to say, "to grow like kudzu," the invasive and ubiq-
uitous vine that grows wild all over the South. The thinking was
that while kids with type 1 could never take a vacation from their
disease, Camp Kudzu could provide them with a fun and healthy
environment, a place where they could learn, grow, and have fun
with other type 1 kids.

Working at Camp Kudzu, in Cleveland, Georgia, that summer
turned out to be one of the best weeks of my life. The kids, who
ranged in age from eight to eighteen, were terrific. We were all out
there in the country, with no e-mails, no phones, just a bunch of

young people (who happened to have diabetes) having a wonderful time together. There was biking, swimming, softball, dancing, and, the favorite of my group of boys, dodgeball. They loved to try to nail me, but as I was not all that older than they were, I still had the dexterity to escape their missiles. There was also some serious stuff—a lot of talking about managing our diabetes—and I was soon having discussions with these kids similar to those I'd had with Joe. I met a couple of kids who were having trouble with the whole issue of being diabetic, and I spent a little more time with them. They left, I think, feeling a little better about themselves than when they had come—and not just because of me but because of the whole positive atmosphere of Camp Kudzu. These kids and I, as well as the other counselors and I, were all connected in a way that even most of my closest buddies couldn't understand. We shared the reality of having a disease that never went away, never went into remission, never let you live a day without making its presence felt.

Yet, we didn't really view it as a struggle. Sure, there were issues that some of these adolescents had to work out (what adolescent doesn't have issues to work out?), but no one was moaning about being a diabetic. Yes, we shared something similar: our pancreases were malfunctioning. But despite that, we were living our lives, feeling good, having fun. Being diabetic united us, but it didn't define us.

While at Kudzu, I talked up our involvement with RAAM and continued to speak in local schools, camps, bike shops, clubs, and, most critically, the offices of potential sponsors. I tried to paint as dramatic a picture as possible. "Do you want to be part of a great adventure, something that will change the perception of diabetes around the world?"

It started to click. I raised enough money to pay my travel to Las Vegas for the Interbike Trade Show, which was for all the bike and equipment manufacturers. A day or two before I left for Vegas, I dropped into Georgia CycleSport in Athens: this was a place I'd known for years, and the manager, Micah Morlock, was a good guy. I was selling life insurance at this point—a junior agent for MassMutual—and had my suit and tie on. I also had my funding proposal for Team Type 1 and our participation in Race Across America. I was looking for $250,000 and product. A couple of guys from the bike-racing crowd were hanging out there that day, and they wanted to see the proposal. I saw them skimming it, and I distinctly remember one guy snickering. "What?" I asked, defensively. "Come on, Junior," he said. "This isn't going to happen. Who the hell is going to give this kind of money to you? I mean, you're a nice guy and all, but really. Two hundred fifty grand? So you and a couple of other guys can ride a bike across the country with those nuts?"

I got mad. "You wait," I said. "You wait and see." I stormed out, determined to get that money and prove him wrong.

Interbike attracts about twelve thousand people every year. In 2005, I was determined to try to meet every one of them—or at least the ones who would help us. I walked the floor of the show, armed with thirty fancy brochures I'd printed up at Kinko's to give out to high-end sponsors, then one hundred black-and-white versions for the smaller vendors. I shook hands and told the story of Team Type 1 and RAAM about five hundred times in the next twenty-four hours. I was walking around in a suit and tie in a sea of bike shorts and T-shirts (it's a casual show). I would have preferred the shorts and T-shirt, but I had to let everybody know that we meant business.

Out of about 500 people that I spoke to, 499 said, "Yes, we'll sponsor your team." When I got back to Atlanta, those 499 turned into a total of 6 people who responded to my follow-up e-mails and phone calls. Five of them were kind enough to donate tires, helmets, wheels, glasses, energy bars, and food. The last one turned out to be the guy who had said no to me in Las Vegas—Herbert Krable of Litespeed, a high-end racing-bike manufacturer. He called me out of the blue and said, "Phil, I want to sponsor your team." He donated thirteen high-end bikes—a retail value of roughly eighty-five thousand dollars.

We had bikes to ride! Now we needed people to help us get across the country—a couple of dozen, at least. We began networking, posting messages on every cycling and diabetes Web site we knew. Slowly but surely it started to work. E-mails began coming in from diabetics and their family members around the country who wanted to help. RAAM is a labor-intensive event. Besides the cyclists themselves, a complete support crew is needed. That means a team of drivers, mechanics, navigators, cooks, and water handlers, all willing to take more than two weeks out of their lives to drive rather slowly across the country. Within days, we had received more than one hundred e-mails—out of which we got our riders, our crew, thousands of dollars of donations, and the support of a lot people with diabetes. I was overwhelmed.

Still, while the ten-dollar individual contributions and best-wishes e-mails were gratifying, we were going to incur some big bills in order to do RAAM. Getting thirty-eight people and a bunch of bicycles across the country ain't cheap. To do it, we'd need vehicles, including two RVs. We'd also require the accoutrements that we diabetics need just to survive. I had an idea about who could provide all that.

At about the same time, I visited my new endocrinologist, Dr.

Bruce Bode. I had met Bruce at Camp Kudzu. He was the pre-
eminent endocrinologist in the Southeast and one of the country's
leading diabetes experts. Bruce was in demand—he had a six-
month waiting list for new patients—but when I mentioned that I
needed a new endocrinologist now that I was no longer living in
Tallahassee, he got me in within a few weeks. While he, like Nancy
Wright, was impressed with how I had managed my diabetes, there
was also a concern. I was having too many low-blood-sugar (hypoglycemic) episodes. He put me in a clinical study for the new Free-
Style Navigator, a continuous glucose-monitoring system by Abbott
Labs that was awaiting approval by the FDA. The system was a
godsend. It constantly fed back to me information on my blood
sugar highs and lows, eliminating the need for me—or any other
diabetic—to have to whip out a blood sugar meter every couple of
hours. The system was particularly valuable for an endurance athlete who would need to know precisely what his levels were while,
say, riding across the country on a bike. Ten days later, I came back
to Dr. Bode for a follow-up appointment. I showed him the device.
"Bruce," I said, "my team has to have this device to win the race.
Who do I talk to at Abbott?"

A few weeks later, I picked up the phone to call Bruce's contact
at Abbott Laboratories, one of the world's largest pharmaceutical
companies and a leader in the development and marketing of
drugs and other products for diabetics. I cold-called their headquarters in Alameda, California. I had a name—Holly Kulp, vice
president of marketing, in charge of marketing and a friend of
Bruce's. Still, I was transferred around and around the vast headquarters. Each time, I had to repeat my quick spiel ("I'm Phil
Southerland, a type 1 diabetic, and I've organized a team of other
type 1 diabetic cyclists who plan to ride across America. We're hoping Abbott can help . . ."). Eight weeks after my last checkup with

Bruce, I found myself in a conference call with two marketing directors who worked under Holly. At the end of it, I was invited to come out to California and make the pitch in person.

On January 25, 2006 I flew to California. This was a day I'll remember for the rest of my life. Nervous and new to the world of business travel and corporate sponsorship, I got out of the plane in Oakland, hopped into a cab (at twenty-four, I still wasn't old enough to rent a car in California) and was driven directly to Alameda. With my suitcase in hand, I walked right into Abbott's massive headquarters and announced to the people at the front desk that I was there. They looked puzzled. A few minutes later, an administrative assistant came out to reception, greeted me, and politely told me that the meeting was not for two more hours. In my excitement, I'd forgotten to adjust for the time difference.

I left, checked in to my hotel, and returned at the appointed time, more nervous than before—but confident that, if given the opportunity, I could persuade them to support us. I was escorted into a conference room. In came four Abbott executives, Steve Bubrick, Curt Jennewine, Mirasol Panlilio and their boss, Holly Kulp, senior vice president of marketing, whose primary responsibility at that point was Abbott's new FreeStyle Navigator, a product that was about to revolutionize diabetic monitoring.

I saw looks of surprise register on their faces when they saw me. Steve chuckled. "Wow," he said. "This isn't what we were expecting." Momentarily flustered—were my socks mismatched? my hair out of place?—I realized what they meant. They had assumed that the founder of Team Type 1 would be a guy around forty, or certainly someone with a little more maturity than the boy who sat waiting for them. Someday, when I'm older, if I have retained my so-called boyish looks, I'll probably be happy about it. But when you're twenty-four and you look sixteen, it's not always a good thing. I didn't wait for them to decide they'd made a mistake. I launched right into my pitch.

I told them again about my team, about RAAM, about how we wanted to show what diabetics could do. I explained what we needed to make this happen. I told them we'd already received significant product sponsorship from the cycling industry. What I would need to cover everything else was... oh, about $140,000. Give us that, I said, and we'll win RAAM.

This was a big number, and I knew it. I braced myself for peals of laughter or a polite but fast exit to the door. Instead, they nodded politely.

I continued, and talked about the FreeStyle Navigator, what a great product it was and how we needed these to monitor our blood sugar across the country. I promised plenty of exposure for the new product: we would ride with the Navigator on our arms, along with the logo on our jerseys and team vehicles. We would use RAAM to promote this important new product, which continuously measures glucose levels through a sensor placed just under the skin in the back of the upper arm or abdomen. The sensor readings are transmitted to a pager-size receiver that displays the glucose levels every sixty seconds. This helps people like me who want to "tightly manage" our disease.

At this point I handed out the proposals I'd photocopied at my local Kinko's and inserted into nice, little plastic binders. "There are 18 million diabetics in America," I said, using the latest statistics at the time, as they followed along. "There are also about 18 million recreational cyclists. Each of those 36 million has an average family size of about 2.75. That's a total audience of 99 million—99 million people that will hear about FreeStyle Navigator!"

Finally, I told them I needed a commitment right away. "I need to know *now* if we can do this," I said dramatically.

The three of them smiled. "We'll get back to you in a week," said Steve. "It looks really promising, and thanks for coming out to meet us in person."

It sounded good, but I wasn't sure. When I got back to my hotel, the phone rang. It was Holly's secretary, Jessica Bloat. She told me that Holly and her husband would like to have dinner with me that night. *Nice gesture,* I thought. *Hope he's not a boring corporate suit or some West Coast flake.*

When we got to the restaurant that evening, Holly introduced me to her husband, Geoff, and told me he was the chemist behind the glucose-monitoring system. I was shocked. This was the guy who had, essentially, invented the first blood-glucose strip, which allows us diabetics to easily and effectively keep track of our glucose levels. Without that, we're dead. I was in awe of meeting the guy who helped keep me, and millions of other diabetics, alive. He turned out to be not at all the way I had expected. He was funny, engaging, and as passionate about fighting diabetes as I was. He had two daughters from a previous marriage, both of whom were also type 1. So we connected well. Holly was also warm and genuine, not at all the arm's-length corporate type that I might have expected from an executive in a major corporation. We talked and talked into the evening about the disease, about the challenges and the breakthroughs. Geoff had heard about my team and our RAAM quest, and we discussed that further.

As the evening wound down, Holly put down her dessert fork, cast her eyes down as if to summon the right words, and then looked at me. "Phil," she said, "finding the money you're asking is going to be tough." My heart sank. *Oh no,* I thought. *What a way to end this wonderful evening. With a punch to the stomach.* Then I heard the "but."

"But Geoff and I have been fortunate in our lives. We've decided what you're doing is so monumental for diabetes that if I can't find money within Abbott, we'll write you a personal check for this race."

I think I must have just sat there staring at her, mouth agape, for a full minute—probably looking like a character from a Warner Bros. cartoon whose jaw unhinges and falls off from shock.

Holly smiled, to make sure I understood. "Your team will do this race."

After hugs and backslaps and handshakes, I raced back to my hotel. It was about nine o'clock—midnight back home. I didn't care. I was crying tears of joy. Phones were soon ringing from Tallahassee to Atlanta. "We're going to do it!" I screamed. "Team Type 1 is a go for RAAM!" I was grateful, but I couldn't help feeling a little sense of vindication. So many people had told me that this was all a pipe dream. "Great idea, but you're not going to get anyone to give you this money" was a refrain I'd heard from a number of people. *Ha!* I thought as I finally lay down to try to rest my jangled, jet-lagged body before the flight home the next day. "Proved you wrong," I said out loud, visualizing the face of the marketing guy at the bike company, the know-it-all friend, and, just for a moment, the physician that had told my mom years earlier that I'd probably be blind or even dead by now. "Proved you wrong."

Today, we have 101 riders on Team Type 1, sixty of whom have type 1 diabetes and twenty-four who have type 2. But in 2005, it was pretty much Joe and I—and he was still finishing up at Auburn at the time. So rounding up the team was my job. In order to show-case as many diabetic cyclists as possible and to include at least one female rider, we had decided to enter the eight-person-team category. Now we had to fill those slots. It was a tall order. We needed riders who could hold it together not only on the bike but in conversations with doctors, reporters, or curious spectators along the way. After all, we weren't just going to race across America; we were going to race to *reach* America, as well, with our message of hope and inspiration.

I was looking for fast cyclists with diabetes—and I was looking for good ambassadors. Through an article in *Diabetes Positive,* I began to locate them.

One of our most important "finds" was Pratt Rather, among the most accomplished diabetic athletes in America. At forty, Pratt was sixteen years older than I at the time, a good cyclist with one particularly important credential on his riding résumé: eleven years earlier, in 1995, he had been on a first-place team in the four-person, mixed-team category at the Race Across America. He was already a RAAM winner; he would know what had to be done.

Besides me, Pratt, and my buddy Joe, there were five others. They came from various backgrounds; some had been diagnosed as diabetics in their teens, others as adults. Their cycling backgrounds varied, too. Several had completed Ironman-distance triathlons, others were competitive local riders. When I look back today on what each of them wrote on our Web site about advice they'd give to others diabetics, I'm still moved and inspired:

STEVE HOLMES, a rider from England who had been diagnosed—and given one year to live—at age twenty-seven. (At the time of 2006 RAAM he was thirty-five, so he'd already beat the odds.)

Steve's advice to other diabetics: "Train hard, be focused, relax and know that you are in control of your diabetes and your future. Your life is yours to make and enjoy every single day. Share your knowledge, wisdom and understanding of the disease with other people, diabetic or not, so everyone knows we do everything we want because we are able to."

TROY WILLARD, thirty-two, a special-education teacher from Augusta, Georgia: "Once you accept what you've been given, you can move on and focus on a healthy life. Diabetes has been the driving force that keeps me going daily. Think of it as a competition, only you are always the leader and can control the outcome."

BOBBY HEYER, forty-one, the CEO of a technology firm in Seattle: "I am inspired and motivated by peers who test the boundaries that others impose. My dreams are made possible by those countless other diabetics. I have a lot to prove, primarily to myself. *I do, to prove I can!*"

JAY HEWITT, thirty-eight, an attorney from Greenville, South Carolina, and an Ironman triathlete: "I accept my diabetes, but I will not surrender to it."

LINDA DEMMA, our other big find: a twenty-nine-year-old woman with a degree from Cornell University and a number of Ironman finishes under her belt: "Try not to let diabetes slow you down—it shouldn't slow you down and it won't. However, be strong enough to admit when you need help, a shoulder to cry on."

For Team Type 1, the shoulders that supported us belonged to our support crew. To find these people, the unsung volunteers who would fix our flats, feed us our meals, plot our course, and essentially hold our hands, as well as our bikes, all the way across the country, I started to reach out to people that I knew. One of the first calls I made was to Ray McNamara, my old Revolutions riding buddy. I told Ray what we were planning to do and how I needed someone I could trust to help out on the crew. Ray may be an ornery character, but he is true blue. He agreed immediately to help out, although later he admitted that he had no idea what he was getting into. "I had heard of RAAM," Ray said, "but I really didn't grasp what it was all about. I think a lot of us who got involved thought we'd be camping out, seeing the country, staying at hotels, and waving at Phil and his team as they rode by. That wasn't the case by a long shot."

In early June 2006—just a little over a year since we'd sat around the table at the Best Western in Carmel, California and decided to do it—the Team Type 1 RAAM team gathered at the San Diego airport. There were a total of thirty-eight—thirty crew and eight riders, including Joe and me. We'd come from all over and had with us all kinds of people, from RAAM-tested veterans like Pratt Rather to my mom and Joe's dad, Dave Eldridge, a building contractor from Birmingham, Alabama, who knew little about cycling and nothing about RAAM, but were always ready to support their sons.

Dave, for one, enjoyed the show that we were about to stage. "It's a full-blown rock concert," he cracked, when he arrived and saw what was going to be involved.

He was right. We were ready to rock. With the sponsor money (which, I was happy to learn, Holly eventually found within Abbott's marketing budget), Pratt had rented two luxury RVs and two cars for the race. Along with our Litespeed Blade TT bikes and Sienna Road bikes—which probably totaled about eighty-five thousand dollars—we were ready to ride and drive the roads of America in style.

The first leg of our journey was to Oceanside, California, about thirty minutes up I-5 from San Diego. When we arrived, there was a real buzz around our team. The blog I had started was getting more and more hits. By race day, there were six thousand to seven thousand people a day reading what we had to say. And what I was saying about RAAM was that we were in it to win it. The media picked up on that boast. There was a photo in an online cycling publication, Pez, a couple of days before the race, showing me looking cocky and confident, flashing a thumbs-up. NEW JERSEY HERE WE COME! said the headline.

We had trained countless hours for this for more than a year and had assembled a team of very experienced, very fit competitive bike riders. To my chagrin, though, no one really seemed to pick up on that. The angle of much of the coverage and much of the feedback I got from other riders and officials at RAAM was, "Wow, it's great what you guys are doing." They might as well have been patting me on the head while they said it. We were stereotyped the way many athletes with disabilities or illnesses are, particularly in participatory sports such as biking, running, and triathlon. After a while I could pretty much fill in the thought balloons over these people's heads. "Oh, look at these heroic young people, courageously struggling to get themselves across the finish line, in order to raise money for their cause. How inspiring!" Don't get me wrong: while we appreciated the good wishes and realized that they were usually genuine, something in that attitude rankled me, and still does. We're athletes, dammit, and we want to be accorded the same respect as other competitors. That's how you treat somebody with illness or disability, in my opinion. Not as a special-needs person, but as a *person*.

At RAAM, we were not just "hoping to finish"—although in an event like RAAM, anyone who finishes is indeed worthy of respect. We were going into this in order to win the damn thing. Specifically, we wanted to be the first team to cross the line. To help ensure that, we entered the so-called Corporate division, which allowed us to field eight riders. Thinking that eight pairs of legs are better than four or two, we figured that was our best chance not only to achieve that goal but to do it faster than anyone in the past. Imagine: a team of diabetics winning a race across the country in record-breaking time! We felt we could, even if nobody else did.

While we knew where we wanted to finish in RAAM, we came perilously close to not even starting. RAAM has some very specific safety rules about bikes used in the race—what kind of lights you needed, where you had to have reflective tape, and so forth. While we were in San Diego, our chief mechanic, Chris Slaton (another old buddy from Tally), realized that we didn't have the right lights on our Litespeeds. "I went driving all over San Diego looking for bike lights," Chris recalls. "I finally found them at the only bike store that was still open. We ended up spending five hundred dollars for them. It became a big scramble. We were very green. It was all new to us, and we had to learn quick."

Once we had arrived in Oceanside, Chris discovered another problem: competitors in RAAM use carbon wheels on their bikes. These are bike wheels that have tubes sewn into the tires, which are then glued to the rim. We didn't have them, which meant we would have to glue each of our tubes to the rim by hand. That process typically takes about two hours per tire. "Wow," Chris told me when he learned of this. "We should have been here three weeks ago." Then, the whole crew had to spring into tire-changing mode. Luckily, a new two-sided adhesive tape had just come out that cut the operation down to five minutes per tire. Chris was able to get some, so, over the course of one night, in their adjoining hotel rooms, he and the other mechanics had a tire-gluing party and had our bikes up to RAAM code, ready to roll.

The teams at RAAM start two days after the solo riders. So those road warriors were already well on their way to the finish line in Atlantic City, New Jersey, when the gun went off for us at 2:00 P.M. Pacific Time, on June 13, 2006. As spectators cheered, Team Type 1 and about thirty other teams rolled down the famous Oceanside Pier, escorted by police up the Strand and onto the San Luis Rey Bike Path. It was some procession: Once we hit the road, each rider and team had an RV ahead of him and a "follow car" behind. Once a rider got going, the van would drive ahead to get the next team rider ready for his "hand off." Joe's dad sat in our follow car, with the 166-page, spiral-bound RAAM Route Book in his hands. We'd hooked up a microphone system so that he could yell out directions to us. "Off we went, on our way from California to Atlantic City, at an average speed of twenty-two miles per hour," he recalls now with a laugh. "All the way with my amplified voice saying, 'Make a left here, make a right there.'"

It would be Dave's job to tell us which way to go for three thousand miles. It was our job to put our heads down and pedal. Our first stage, fifty-four miles, took us from Oceanside along lightly traveled roads into the shadow of Palomar Mountain (site of the famous observatory) near the crest of the Laguna Coastal ranges. My first shift was almost all uphill. It was hard, but I was fired up, knowing we were here and finally on the move as a team. I realized we still had three thousand miles to go, but I was confident in my teammates and our crew.

That confidence was shaken the first night, when my friend Tim Henry—who was handling our nutrition—made an understandable but serious error. After we'd completed our first eight-hour shift, the four of us on Type 1's A-team—Joe, Bobby Heyer, Jay Hewitt, and I—went to sleep after drinking our recovery drink. We took our shots, seven to ten units of insulin, to compensate for the amount of carbohydrate we thought were in the drink: 130 grams.

Quick lesson in diabetic biochemistry: insulin lowers blood sugar, food raises it. So if you take one unit for fifteen grams of carbohydrate, and get only one-quarter of the amount of carbs, your blood sugar is going in one direction—down, down, to dangerous, hypoglycemic levels.

An hour after we'd gone to sleep, all these beeps starting going off in the van. We wake up and realize it's our FreeStyle Navigators telling us that our blood sugar is low. We all grab something to eat, go back to sleep. A little while later, the Navigators start beeping again. Still low. We kept eating and taking glucose tabs and finally we get back up to normal. Because we were highly insulated and undercarbed, we could have gone into hypoglycemic shock. We would have, if not for the Navigators, which proved their value, and not just because of the sponsorship money they represented. The next morning, we were still trying to figure out what had happened when I noticed Tim making drinks to hand out to the riders. I told him he was putting in only one scoop instead of four. "Oh, man," he said. "Sorry, I read the label wrong."

I begged him not to make the mistake again, please. He didn't. As I jokingly tell people to this day, we're still friends, even though he tried to kill me.

Seriously, if one of us had gone into hypoglycemic shock or died that night in the Mojave Desert, it would have been more than just a human tragedy. It would have been a big story—and a big loss for people with diabetes. Our attempt to do RAAM, Team Type 1, and our basic mission—to show that people with diabetes are capable of doing anything anyone else is, provided they take care of themselves—that all would have died, too.

While we were having our drama that night, the other Team Type 1 foursome had been forging ahead. That was according to plan. Although we would be scored as an eight-person team, we had divided our riders into two groups of four. Each team would be self-sustaining, with their own RVs and support crews. One crew would ride while the other would sleep. Team Type 1 would become a nonstop operation.

Timing was everything here. In relay races on the track, one runner hands a baton to the next. In RAAM, team transitions are more complex and potentially dangerous, particularly at night on open roads. Four pages in the RAAM guidebook are devoted to what is and what it isn't a legal or safe transition, what the bikes and vehicles have to do, how far and how fast, where they can stop, and so forth. Essentially, the transition occurs when the new racer overlaps wheels with the racer he or she is replacing. The new rider can either stop and wait for that to occur—that is, sit still on his bike until the rider on the previous leg has pulled up beside him—or he can make the exchange with the new rider already rolling. Naturally, because every second counted for us, we chose the latter. We would do that over and over and over—each of us riding for a fifteen-to-twenty-minute "pull," as we called it, transitioning to the next guy, who would ride for twenty minutes, so on and so on for hours. While you're riding, one van would scoot ahead to get the next rider and his bike ready. Of course, someone had to make sure we were on course the whole time.

The RAAM course is divided into fifty-seven sections, with so-called time-reporting stations every thirty-five to eighty miles. These stations, manned by local volunteers, are located near convenience stores or gas stations, some in the middle of substantial communities, others in little crossroads settlements. The route itself sounds like a Johnny Cash song: Salton City, Prescott, Flagstaff, Durango, Alamosa, Montezuma. At the end, I could truly say, "I've been everywhere, man." But as our little caravan rolled slowly across the continent, our main focus was not on the scenery—as magnificent as it was—but on getting ready for our pulls and trying to adjust to living in a crowded RV. There were five of us in one. When it was our turn to sleep, we shared beds. Conditions got bad; the RV was really not built to handle so many of us, and very quickly the toilet got clogged up, the interior got dirty, it was pretty crummy. Still, the mood stayed good. I had Joe, Bobby Heyer, and Jay Hewitt in my van. We were constantly making fun of one another, trying to stay loose. Jay didn't know us that well, and he was a little tense the first couple of days. I wasn't helping things: every time he'd ride, I'd lean out the van window and yell, "Get in your drops, get in your drops!" I was referring to the lower parts of the drop handlebar—shaped like a horizontal U—on a racing bike. You go into your drops to help make yourself lower and more aerodynamic. Right before Durango, Colorado, 815 miles and three days into the race, as Jay was just getting started on a pull, he looked up at me as the van came by. "If you tell me to get in my drops I'm going to break your neck," he growled. Everybody howled with laughter. Jay was out of his shell, and from then on, we were a unit.

As we chugged along, we must have looked like something out of *The Road Warrior,* a movie about a nomadic group of survivors in a postapocalyptic world. Often, we were alone for miles and miles, moving through the desert at twenty-five miles an hour, one van festooned with five bikes on the roof, a pace car zipping up ahead, music blasting over the speakers, and one tired rider pedaling away behind. Every eight hours, we would see the other half of our team—Pratt, Linda, Steve, and Troy—for five minutes. We'd say hello, you're doing great, but they ended up being almost like a separate team, even though our results counted together. A few days into the race, it became apparent that splitting the team into two had been a mistake—mine alone. Instead of two parts of a whole working toward the same goal, we became rivals in our little competition—and not in a healthy way. There was some childish behavior, some snickering and teasing of the other team's efforts that at the time was meant to be funny, but really wasn't. It didn't help their morale, and although they rode their hearts out, too, they didn't feel appreciated. They should have been, and the appreciation for their outstanding efforts should have come from me, the team leader. It didn't, and I regret that now.

Instead of petty infighting between the two Teams Type 1, the ones we really should have been worrying about were the team called Vail Beaver Creek. Here, my cockiness and confidence in my teammates came back to haunt me. This four-man group from Vail, Colorado, had won the team race on two previous occasions. They were professionals—at this point, we weren't—but they were mountain bikers. They rode the heavier, fat-tire cycles for a living. Despite the fact that I'd started out as a mountain biker as a kid, I'd long since become a skinny-tire snob. Like a lot of road-bike racers, I tended to look down at the mountain bikers as guys who rode over logs and on trails. Impressive in its own way, but not "real" bike racing. Plus, there were four of them and eight of us.

Our coach, Rick Crawford, knew them and had told me before the start, "Phil, you better watch out for those Vail guys." I dismissed it. "How fast can mountain bikers be?" I replied.

He said, "Fast. Very fast." I saw how right he was when the Vail Creek guys took a very fast and early lead against us. Right away we were behind, and I was pissed. I wanted us to be the first team across America—and I certainly didn't want our eight beaten by their four.

The key moment came at Wolf Creek Pass in Colorado. This is a key point in RAAM for many reasons. They call it a "working-man's climb," and they're right about the work part—it's tough. The road is an 8 percent grade that doesn't begin to flatten out until you crest at 10,550 feet—which also happens to be the point of the Continental Divide. With two more, slightly less severe but still hard, climbs following it, this is RAAM's Rocky Mountain High.

We were wheezing, panting, dying as we pedaled up those mountains. The Vail team was on their home court. No way could we catch those Colorado mountain bikers in their own mountains. The best we could hope for was not to fall too far behind. Coach Rick had an idea about how do that. "Let's limit our losses by try-ing a new strategy," he said. "Let's do shorter, more intense pulls." In other words, instead of a hard fifteen-to-twenty-minute effort, an all-out, two-to-four-minute effort. That would mean more transitions, and every transition is a bit of a risk. But I liked the idea. "Let's go for it," I said. So we did, for eight hours, transition-ing on and off through the Colorado night. While I was nearly cross-eyed at the end of my last pull, we got to the time station at South Fork, Colorado—the end of that leg—and found that we'd lost only four minutes to the Vail team. We all cheered. That was a big, big boost for us. We'd expected to lose twenty to thirty minutes to the mountain bikers in their mountains. But we'd stayed close.

Now came the Great Plains, where we could show these guys just how fast a bunch of pumped-up diabetics could ride. "The race is on!" I said to my teammates. "We've got half a continent to go. We can catch these guys! Let's do it!"

11

Are You a Bike Rider . . . or a Bike *Racer*?

Just think—the Tour de France is 2178 miles in 3 weeks.
This has been 3060 miles in 5 and ½ days.

—TEAM TYPE 1 RAAM BLOG

The first thousand miles of the 2006 Race Across America, we didn't have a really clear picture of where our blood sugar levels needed to be. No type 1s had ever done anything like this. There were no studies, no consensus statements, no guidelines, no nothing about how to manage diabetes while attempting to race a bicycle across the continent.

After the mountains, I found that when my blood sugar levels were between 140 and 180, I was strong during my pulls—and felt refreshed and ready to go for the next ones. Same with Joe. This was a vital piece of information for all eight of us and we immediately spread the word among our teammates. Working out the diabetes strategy was as important as our race strategy. Bike-racing teams have to worry about a lot of things; Team Type 1 has to worry about all those same things *plus* a potentially life-threatening disease.

Once we'd more or less synchronized our blood sugar targets, I sensed a new air of confidence. We had a tailwind, we were cruising along the highways of the Great Plains at forty miles per hour, and things were looking brighter—for the moment. I remember blasting downhill at one point, maybe hitting forty-five miles per hour, when a violent crosswind buffeted my Litespeed, aerodynamic with its Zipp Wheels. The bike's frame was made from titanium alloy, and true to its name, it weighed only about seventeen pounds. I was blown across the width of a two-lane highway, the gust was so strong. The bike began shaking, and I managed to get my hands on the brakes to slow it down without crashing. I rolled to a stop in a little valley, and the follow car screeched to a stop on the side of the road to make sure I was still upright.

"That was close!" I said. "Where did that wind come from?"

A look at the horizon provided the answer. Dark clouds were gathering in the very direction our vehicles were headed. We were going to be in for a very rough ride. The winds picked up as we continued, the clouds thickening and darkening. On the radio, we began hearing about wind gusts up to sixty-five miles per hour. Then, lightning strikes flashed in the distance.

"Get off your bikes and get in the car!" called Dave Eldridge.

We kept riding, taking our turns on our fifteen-minute pulls. "There's no way that Vail team is stopping, so we can't either," I said. My teammates all agreed.

In retrospect, we probably should have listened to Dave. Soon after we crossed the border into Kansas, we heard on the radio that the storm had knocked down power lines and left the communities around us without electricity. There were cars pulled over along the side of the road. The rain came down in torrents at certain points, the wind rattled the bikes and the vehicles, even our big RV; lightning crisscrossed the sky. It continued that way for an hour and a half, and although we were all terrified, we tried to reassure ourselves (and our worried parents and friends) that we'd be okay.

"We're riding titanium bikes and we're on rubber wheels," I said, sounding more confident than I actually was. "The lightning won't find us."

Of course, I had no way of knowing whether this was true—luckily, the theory was never tested. We covered 250 miles in ten hours that night, and by the time the storm abated, we learned that we had made up an hour on Beaver Creek. Although we never got confirmation, we suspected that they *had* stopped—and if they had, it was because they were saner and smarter than we were. Then again, those guys weren't racing to prove something, the way we were. They were a team of superb riders and fierce competitors who wanted to win the Race Across America. We were riding to make a statement on behalf of 1.5 million people who have a disease that's constantly in their lives, relentless, unceasing, and unforgiving—so how could we be anything but? After the storm, we had the Vail team in our crosshairs, and we were gaining. It was all-out, every time. After each pull, the rider could barely walk and would have to be helped back to the car.

We caught them in Missouri. We were coming out of Jefferson City and had heard that they were just ahead. The gap began to close: Team Type 1 was five miles behind, four miles, three miles, and then we saw a small knot of riders and vehicles moving along the road in the distance. It was exciting: for the first time in days, we felt that we were competing against something other than Mother Nature and the monotony of the highway. Still, our cycling drama played out before an empty house. While there were a few spectators during RAAM, and many communities along the way came out to welcome and support us as we rumbled through, most people across this vast land of ours had no idea that a bike-racing caravan was coming through their town. Our cat-and-mouse game with the Vail team played out on a very lonely stretch of the Great American Highway.

That was okay, though: we didn't need a live audience. There was no Twitter yet to allow us to keep our fans posted on a minute-by-minute basis, but we did have our friends and family members, the folks at Abbott, people we knew from Camp Kudzu and the JDRF, and others, all tracking our progress and spreading the word, via e-mail and Web site posts, around the diabetes community. We began getting e-mails of best wishes from complete strangers, people saying prayers for us, parents wishing us Godspeed and telling us how what we were doing was inspiring their diabetic child.

I also recall looking around at one point and thinking that while I was a man who was doing a lot of suffering on the road, I was a very lucky man, at that. One of my teammates was my best friend; our crew chief was his dad; our photographer and webmaster was my mom; and three of the friends I'd had for more than a decade—Chris, Ray and Michael Scholl—were an integral part of my support team. They were all there because of me. Admittedly, in part because I'd cajoled them to be there, but they all did it on their own volition, because they believed in me and our cause and in Team Type 1. It was a humbling realization.

It was also somewhat chaotic. We were really making this up as we went along, which is probably typical of most of the teams and riders who do RAAM for the first time. I mean, think about it: what really prepares you to organize something like this? I knew in the back of my mind that there were ways we could improve the efficiency. At one point, Ray came up to me and for once didn't offer me a good-natured razzing. "Phil," he said, "now is not the time, I know, but once this is over, I have some ideas on how we could make this operation more efficient."

I was impressed that Ray was thinking about the next time—in part because several times a day, when my quads burned and my entire body screamed "Enough!" I really wasn't sure there would be a second time for this, no matter what the outcome.

The moment we took the lead wasn't like some decisive attack in a Tour de France stage that makes the highlight reels. In a race like that, you don't have to worry about where you're going. The course is well marked, and besides, you're in a pack of a hundred or so other riders. RAAM is different. Half the battle is knowing where you are. This wasn't like my nearly straight-line solo ride from Athens to Tally, where I'd had to make only a dozen or so turns the whole route. Each team in RAAM is issued a route book with 145 pages of directions and course descriptions to follow, as detailed as this section, between Jefferson City and Marthasville, Missouri.

Turn right, U.S. 54 E on ramp (immediately after small local street), do not cross over U.S. 54

Yield: merge to rejoin 54 E

Cross Missouri River

Stay on US 54 E toward Mokane, Do Not Exit to Airport

Right Exit 3 off ramp toward SR/Mokane . . . merge onto SR 94 E at "Yield"

Cross Logan Crk, begin 8 mi. of short steep windy rollers, 5 exceeding 100'

Portland: Yield one lane bridge

Right junct hwy D, turn to stay on SR 43, toward Rhineland

It goes on like that for . . . well, an entire continent. As specific and careful as those directions are, is it any wonder that someone could make a wrong turn here or there over the course of three thousand miles? That's what happened to our rivals from Vail, at a bad time for them. There was this road that wasn't well marked. But we had a good navigator in Dave Eldridge, who saw the sign and yelled, "Right, right." Our rider made the right. The Vail guys had missed the sign, kept on going straight, and got caught at a railroad crossing. We were close enough to see them, so we honked the horn of our lead vehicle and hoped they would see us making the right turn. (It was the sportsmanlike thing to do.)

Our lead was temporary. I was out on a pull with Joe when one of their guys caught up with us at a stop light. We exchanged some pleasantries. I told them how much fun it was racing them, and what a great event this was. The light turned green and this guy from Vail attacked like it was the first lap of Athens Twilight. Joe and I looked at each other and then started chasing him. We were gaining at the next intersection. But he caught the green, and we got stuck on the red, and waited. And waited. It was a three-minute red light in the middle of rural Missouri! Not a single car passed—but still, one of the many rules of RAAM is that you can't run a red light no matter what. We sat there and watched our opponent disappear in the distance.

My heart sank at that moment. It seemed that as soon as we'd had the lead, it was gone. But fortunes change quickly over the length of America, as ours did about two states, and two hundred miles farther down the road. By then it was night and were coming out of Indianapolis. We were doing forty miles per hour on pitch-black roads, and around a bend, there they were. A lone cyclist on the road, a pair of headlights illuminating from behind. It was during one of Joe's pulls, and he soared past them. Over the next eighty miles, we opened a ten-to-fifteen-minute gap.

That, it turned out, was the decisive move for us in RAAM 2006. Still, we knew that we were racing a bunch of professional mountain-bike riders. To make sure that we would maintain our lead, we decided over the last twenty-seven hours of the race to do shorter and shorter pulls to keep up the average speed. What was already grueling and difficult became downright torture—almost a flat-out sprint every time you got on the bike, which you kept doing, it seemed, again and again and again. And with less sleep. I'd ride my pull, get into the car, and immediately fall asleep. Someone would shake me: "Phil, it's your turn." I'd wake up and get right back on the bike (we slept in spandex), ride full throttle for another four to five miles, then collapse again. I felt like a ping-pong ball, bouncing from feeling dead tired to nearly killing myself with effort. It was hell. Still, we held on to our lead, or so we thought.

Along with 145 pages of directions, the RAAM Route Guide also features about forty pages of rules. That wasn't always the case. When the race started, the rules were few. But over the years, the number of regulations grew with the success of the event. Most of them have to do with support vehicles on the course, which runs through fourteen states and 350 communities. "We couldn't have a race if we had to get permits from every single one of them," says RAAM president Fred Boethling. "So we operate essentially at the pleasure of the administrative bodies along the way." Having lanes blocked by support vehicles—which could prompt calls from angry motorists and local constituents—is not likely to endear RAAM to these administrative bodies. "We have to keep them happy," Boethling admits. Hence, the rules.

At that point in the 2006 race, all I wanted was to see that finish-line banner on the boardwalk at Atlantic City. With forty miles to go, we put all four of our riders on the road—a sort of mass attack. Joe, Bobby, Jay, and I sprinted under the banner at thirty-five miles per hour. Then we whooped and hollered. We congratulated ourselves on winning the 2006 Race Across America.

There was just one problem:

We hadn't won.

A half hour after we'd crossed the line—and completed the ceremonial winner's "victory lap" along the boardwalk—an official came over to us. "Sorry guys," he said. "Vail won by three minutes."

In seconds, my mood went from elation to shock and dejection. I don't think I've ever been more disappointed in my life, than that day on the boardwalk at Atlantic City.

Later, it was explained to me that we had broken several of the RAAM rules, including the "caravanning" rule, where support vehicles are prohibited from lining up behind the follow vehicle, clogging up a lane. As a result, we'd been assessed a fifteen-minute penalty.

"We kept getting sketchy information on the course," Chris recalls. "At one point, we had been told we had three penalties, which would have totaled an hour and a half. Yet somehow, at the end, I guess we only had the one, for fifteen minutes. The reasons we had been given were caravanning, too many cars together with the racer at one time, running a stop sign, and leaving course and reentering at a different location. I never did hear which one stuck."

Conflicting recollections of exactly what happened are not uncommon in a sleep-deprivation endurance event like RAAM. "I raced the 2006 race," says Boethling, "and my memories are at times distinctly different from those of my crew!"

I was vaguely aware of the penalties, but they'd happened earlier in the race and I guess I never really thought they would impact the final standing. Besides, I was too focused on getting the blood sugars right, getting through each pull, and catching the Vail team. But, as it turned out, we paid a huge price for those infractions.

Deducting the fifteen-minute penalty put us three minutes behind the Vail team. The final results:

Beaver Creek-Vail: *5 days, 16 hours, 1 minute (average speed: 22.37 mph)*

Team Type 1: *5 days, 16 hours, 4 minutes (average speed: 22.36 mph)*

To think that we'd crossed an entire continent and only three minutes separated us. Still, we had to keep it in perspective. In RAAM 2006 there were twenty solo racers (twenty-seven men and two women) and twenty-eight teams (of two, four, and eight riders, plus a six-person hand-cycle team). That's a total of 143 competitors. We'd won the eight-person-team competition. The guys from Beaver Creek won the four-person and were the first team across the line. When you think about it, four guys who could give eight guys such a race over 3,042.8 miles probably deserved the overall team win, anyway.

Second, our real goal in competing in RAAM was to show something about what diabetics—properly trained and carefully monitoring their blood sugar—could do. In that contest, we'd broken no rules, and perhaps we'd written a few new ones.

At the moment I heard about our reverse, however, I wasn't feeling so magnanimous. As we milled about the boardwalk, in a state of shock and exhaustion, I swore that we'd never do RAAM again. Then my cell phone rang. It was Steve Bubrick, by then director of marketing at Abbott Diabetes Care. "Phil, from all of us at Abbott, I want to give you a huge thank-you," he said. "What you've done has been so inspiring. We are floored. Amazing, amazing, amazing. Now, I have a question for you."

What's that?

"Would you be willing to do it again?"

Less than thirty minutes after we crossed the finish was probably not the best time to ask that question, and I think Steve sensed that. Before I could roar "Hell, no!" he quickly added a few important points.

"Let me make it clear, Phil, that if you do decide to do it again, we would be returning as your sponsor, and I think with an even bigger commitment than this year."

I thought about the errors we'd made out there, the lessons learned. About the organization, about diabetes management, about working with the riders, the crew, not to mention the RAAM rule book. It sure would be nice to go back with some of the same good people I'd just crossed the country with, and correct those errors—maybe with enough money to really do it right.

"I'll do it again, Steve," I said. "But this time . . . we're going to win it. I guarantee you."

My Joe Namath moment over, I repaired to the hotel room we'd prebooked for a hot shower and a nap. But I'd barely gotten into the room when my phone rang again. This time it was Chris, and he sounded concerned. "I'm down here at the storage unit," he said. "What am I supposed to do with all this stuff? No one knows where to put it." We had a trailer full of bikes, wheels, gear, and diabetes supplies, which had been parked right after we finished and was now sitting in a parking garage not far from the finish line. There was probably a hundred thousand dollars' worth of stuff there and it had to get back to Atlanta. Considering that it weighed half a ton, you couldn't very well ask a mailman to deliver it. For once, I didn't have an answer. I'd never really planned past the finish line of the race. What's more, I'd gotten into a fight with the rider who was supposed to have taken care of this, and he had apparently gone home the minute the race was done. How the hell were we going to get all this stuff 670 miles from Atlantic City to Atlanta?

I went down to the parking garage. I must have stood there looking stupefied, which I was, as I had not a clue what to do. Ray came up to me and assessed the situation in his usual, unambiguous terms.

"Phil, you're screwed," he said.

"Thanks, Ray," I said. "I know that, and I'm so tired I can't think straight."

"You want me to help?"

"Yes, please."

"Okay, you got a checkbook?"

"Yes."

"Are you hungry?"

"Starved."

"Great, let's go get something to eat, and I'll tell you what we're going to do."

Over breakfast, Ray told me that instead of hopping on a plane and flying home to Tallahassee the next morning, as most of the rest of the crew would be doing, he and another guy, Matt, would take care of getting the trailer down to Atlanta. The next morning, I had to fill out some forms at the Budget Rental office and sign some checks, almost sleepwalking as I did, but Ray guided me through. Somehow, he and Matt then got everything loaded and packed up and drove the trailer, loaded with all the equipment, all the way home.

Just before he left, Ray also scolded me for not being better organized and for pissing off too many people, in particular the guy who was supposed to have taken care of this. I nodded my head wearily. "But," he added, "you also did something great here."

I smiled, genuinely touched to hear it coming from Ray. He

smiled. "Who would have thought a dumb little Philbert like you could have pulled this off?"

RAAM changed everything. What I'd first picked up during my ride from Athens to Tallahassee—the sense that even people who had not the slightest interest in conventional bike races were intrigued by the idea of someone pedaling down long, lonely highways for hundreds of miles—turned out to be right. Except that after RAAM, it was more than a gaggle of retirees at a McDonald's or a few guys at crossroads convenience store. A few weeks after RAAM, Abbott Diabetes Care invited me to attend the Children with Diabetes Conference in Orlando. I was paid five hundred dollars a day to stand in my spandex bike outfit and talk to kids—something I probably would have done for free, truth be told. A few of them knew who we were. "I read about you in *Diabetes Positive*," one parent told me. "I followed you during the race online," a kid told me. As the buzz spread about the diabetic bike rider who had just raced his bike across the country, lines began forming in front of our booth. Some of the kids were shy, a few wanted my autograph, and others wanted to ask about the race. Most just wanted to talk about how I managed my diabetes. When you're a kid with a disease that your friends don't have, you feel alone, isolated. Oh, sure, you know about what you can do and can't do. You've been warned and lectured by parents, educators, doctors. I was a different person delivering the same message—not an authority figure but someone more like them. I urged them all to try to get their A1c readings under control. The A1c is a common three-month measure of blood sugar—a snapshot of how your diabetes management is going. The ideal A1c reading is 6.5, and this would eventually became a big part of the Team Type 1 message (see "Strive for 6.5," at the end of this book). At the time of the conference, I was just trying to give these kids a simple goal, one that would prod them to start checking their blood sugar a little more regularly, being more aware of their diet, starting to exercise—all the basic things we knew they needed to be doing.

Of course, I also knew these were kids, so any behavioral change had to be approached like a transaction. "What do *you* want?" I'd ask them as part of the A1c pitch. "You give me the 6.5, what do you get? Is there something you'd really like?" They'd say, "A pair of shoes," or, "A new baseball mitt." Then, I'd turn to the parents, who were usually standing right there. "If they get their A1c levels to 6.5, are you okay with getting them that?" They were. As any parent knows, a little bribery often works. Plus, the kids were now accountable; they had this goal, and a reward to look forward to.

It had all been different for me, I realize, growing up in a different era and in different circumstances than many of these kids. When I was young, Joanna couldn't offer me much in the way of reward. Luckily for her, I wanted to control my diabetes and didn't need much incentive (except maybe at Halloween). I simply didn't know another way. Seeing these kids and some of those I'd met at Camp Kudzu the summer before, I began to realize that I was the exception, the anomaly. When it came to taking charge of their disease, many of these kids were AWOL. Some of them were in denial, some of them were a little lazy, and some hoped it would just go away. They needed to learn that their diabetes wasn't going to magically vanish overnight, and that they had to take a greater role in helping themselves. If they did so, they could for the most part live the "normal" lives they craved. As I told them (and continue to tell young diabetics) *wanting* to control your diabetes is half the battle.

We couldn't reach every kid that day, but I know we made an

impression on many of them. I have the Facebook posts and e-mails to prove it. Let me tell you, there was nothing like reading messages six months later from these kids, telling me that their A1c levels had improved and thanking me for talking to them. It was almost as thrilling as winning a bike race.

There was an agent at this conference who (so I was told) represented several diabetic athletes. He walked straight up to the booth like a VIP. "Phil, let's chat," he said. I looked behind him. There were four kids on line waiting to talk to me, and he'd cut ahead of them.

"With all due respect, sir," I said, "you can get in line."

"What?" I could see he was not a man used to hearing the word *no,* especially from diabetics, as if we were supposed to worship him. "I'm here for them," I said, nodding at the kids. "I'll be happy to talk with you another time." He got all hot and walked way. Not for a second did I think I'd made a mistake. I wanted no part of someone who thought he was more important than these type 1 kids.

The conference was a big success for us, and Abbott invited us to another one. That fall, the American Association of Diabetes Educators invited me to speak at their conference. I told them our story—basically connecting some of the "dots" of my life—and it went over big, in part I think because I'm living proof of what these educators were teaching type 1 (and increasingly, type 2) kids. After my talk, a woman attending the conference pulled me aside. "How much did you get paid to speak here?" I told her: five hundred dollars. "You're way better than that," she replied. "You need to get at least two thousand." Hey, I was in sales, I know how to ask for more money. So the next speaking request that came along, I asked for two thousand dollars—and got it! Soon, I had lined up ten to fifteen talks for the next three months. I was sharing the team's message, helping other diabetics, and actually getting paid to do it.

When you consider that a guy who was too shy to interact with most of his high school classmates was now speaking in front of audiences of hundreds of strangers, it's pretty amazing. For some people, public speaking is terrifying—and I suppose if I had to get up in front of a room and talk about the federal budget deficit, or what causes lightning to strike or almost any other topic that I know little or nothing about (of which there are many), I'd be trembling with fear. But I do know about my life and I do know something about diabetes and how to keep it at bay. And that's what I'd talk about, basically covering five or six points, from the fear of blindness, which got me motivated, to my discovery that riding my bike all afternoon allowed me to have a Snickers bar; from the burrito bets with Joe to Team Type 1, RAAM, and our A1c challenge.

Meanwhile, we still had a "real" job to contend with, one that was now conflicting with my outside activities. By now I had been working for MassMutual insurance for about a year. In life insurance sales, the mantra is "take people to lunch, take people to lunch," which is what I was doing. Over lunch, however, the conversation would inevitably turn to Team Type 1 and RAAM. I must admit, potential clients found those subjects far more interesting than my discussion of premiums.

Before long, it got to the point where my heart was no longer in life insurance sales (if it ever really had been in the first place). I left, and with no hard feelings, I might add—my bosses seemed to sense that I had a different calling in life and wished me only the best. I began getting my health insurance through the provisions of the government's Continuous Omnibus Budget Reconciliation Act, known as COBRA for short. It cost me four hundred dollars a month, a huge expense at the time and one that I couldn't really afford. I think of friends of mine in similar situations—young men and women, willing and eager to work hard and take a risk on a new venture, as I was about to do. They couldn't afford health care either, and so for a few years in their twenties and early thirties they would go without, while they built their businesses. I never had such an option. If I didn't have health insurance, I'd be both bankrupt and dead in short order. Just another compromise that a diabetic must make with his or her life.

When it came to Team Type 1, I was now, as the Brits say, in for a penny, in for a pound. I had a ton of work to do. I couldn't do it alone, and my partner was too busy earning a cushy living in construction management. That's what Joe had majored in at Auburn, and now he had landed a job in Memphis that earned him good money, involved little risk, and promised a bright future. The comfortable, safe play for Joe would have been just to stay where he was, which was with a construction firm (not to mention a girlfriend!). I applied all my selling skills to persuade him to take a huge gamble—leave the job and join me to help run Team Type 1, which at that point still consisted of little more than a bank account and a Web site. We talked on the phone every night that spring, sometimes about RAAM and our training but also about his future with Team Type 1.

"I need your help, I need your help," was my refrain every night.

"I don't know, I don't know," was his response.

It was frustrating. I desperately needed help to make Team Type 1 evolve the way I was starting to envision it—as a full-time professional bike-racing team, but also an educational and advocacy group for diabetics. Finally, in May, a month before RAAM, he relented. "All right, man," he said. "I'll do it." Joe gave two weeks' notice and started with Team Type 1. He didn't have a title and his starting salary was zero. The most urgent priority in his job? Help us win the 2007 Race Across America.

Our second time at RAAM, Team Type 1 was no longer a curiosity. We were serious contenders to win, and everyone there knew it. We were also unified in our approach to diabetes. We each knew where our blood sugar needed to be and had the tools to keep it there: FreeStyle Navigators, Omnipods and a Sanofi-Aventis rapid-acting insulin. I was interviewed by local media and recognized by many of the other competitors as well as some of the fans who gathered in Oceanside. Oh yes, and the Beaver Creek boys were back, as well. They knew who we were now, that's for sure. We knew that they were professional bike racers and very good at their job. It was a friendly rivalry, but I was determined that the first bike rider crossing the finish line would be wearing a Team Type 1 jersey.

This time around, we had reason to be confident: We knew the race strategy that could work for us. We also knew that we (especially I, as the team leader) needed to create a more relaxed environment, where everyone felt recognized and appreciated. We had brought too large a crew the year before—a common mistake at RAAM. This time, we cut it down from thirty-five to seventeen, and had a new guy running the show. With Ray McNamara as crew chief, I had a guy I could trust, someone who'd gone through the experience with us the year before but was willing to make changes in order to make it a supertight, efficient operation. Ray could be counted on in a crisis, as he proved by handling the equipment at the end of the 2006 race. I also knew that he would not mince words or sugarcoat anything. If something was going wrong, if I or someone else was screwing up along the way, I'd hear about it from him—in no uncertain terms.

On the first day of the race—June 12, 2007—things got off to a good start when Joe passed a guy from Beaver Creek just a few miles outside of Oceanside. One of their guys passed me in the Laguna Mountains, as I got stung by a bee on my first pull. Then the lead seesawed back and forth. It was one of our new Type 1 riders, Matt Vogel, who made what proved to be the decisive move, less than two hundred miles into the three-thousand-mile race. We were approaching Interstate 10 between Salton City and Chiriaco Summit, in California. There's a rule in RAAM that once you're on an interstate you can't pass another team, for safety reasons. Whoever got on the interstate first, then, would hold the lead for the next ten miles or so. Matt and one of the Beaver Creek guys had an all-out sprint to see who would get to the entry ramp first. Matt just edged him out, we took the lead there, and put twenty minutes on them that night.

Now we were the rabbits, and we had a long way to run. I remember a stretch in Arizona where it was 115 degrees and we had a twenty-four-mile-per-hour headwind. It was like riding with a giant blow dryer in your face. "The desert is not a forgiving environment," we were told in the official course description in our RAAM route book. That's an understatement—and it doesn't apply just to the desert. The mountains, the plains, the prairies— when you're riding for five hours a day for five straight days, there is no forgiveness, no mercy anywhere. RAAM really teaches you how to suffer, and you plumb new bottoms of pain with each hour. Sometimes it's the heat, sometimes it's your body, sometimes it's the slightest imperfection in the transitions.

When you're pulling in RAAM, you're always looking for the van—the one that drives ahead of you, with the next rider—because when you see it pass, you know your pull is almost done. At one point, I was in Monument Valley, Utah, on one of my five-mile pulls, going full gas. At three miles, the van usually passes. I hit three miles, no van. Four miles, no van. I'm at five miles, what should have been the end of my pull, and still no van. Now I'm angry, I'm hot, I'm tired. The follow car pulls up next to me. Where is that van? I ask. They didn't know (turned out, the van driver had pulled over to grab lunch and underestimated the time it would take). So I start slowing down. I've had it. At that point Dave Eldrige leans out the window. "Son," he says, "are you a bike rider or a bike *racer?*"

"I'm a bike *racer,* goddammit," I yell back.

"Well, then show me some attitude and ride like one!"

I did. We all did.

Under the Ray regime, things were far better organized, but conditions became more spartan in order to save time. An example was the showering situation. The first year, we had people changing the water tanks in the RV every eight hours so we'd have hot water. Ray wanted to minimize stops, so I guess you could say we went commando in our showering in 2007. At the end of every shift, you'd get naked, and someone would stand on top of a van and pour water on you for a minute. That was our shower for five days.

Even though we had opened up a good lead, we were always worried about the Beaver Creek riders—particularly in the mountains. Back at Wolf Creek Pass, we went full throttle. I'd never worked as hard in my life as I did there. We had decided to shorten the pulls to two to three minutes, so it was basically a flat-out sprint every time you were on the bike, and at an elevation of eleven thousand feet, you feel like you're breathing through a straw while doing it. The crew on that stage, our buddy Carl Cheshire, and another crew member, Darren, were remarkable—as efficient as a NASCAR pit crew. They had three or four minutes at most to get a rider off his bike and into the van, then put his bike on the roof, drive three-quarters of a mile up the road, and start the process again. They did this with amazing precision, again and again and again.

When we hit the bottom of Wolf Hill Pass, we got the word on our rivals. We were an hour and a half ahead of them. There was no celebrating, because we knew full well that a couple of hours' lead could evaporate quickly, as it had for them the preceding year when we caught up. But we were excited to have the lead and determined to keep it. Again, the drive to prove something larger here, larger than a bike race, was propelling us. There was no way anyone was going to catch us now.

The second half of RAAM 2007 was a race against time—and not just the elapsed time, or the time lead we had over the Beaver Creek team (who, true to form, never gave up and kept the heat on us through the entire Midwest). Rather, we were racing against a *sleep* clock. By cutting our crew in half, we'd gained efficiency and a great camaraderie. But we were now asking people—not just the riders, but the drivers, the handlers, the guys making our meals, reading the maps, and pouring water on our heads—to go well beyond the limits of their endurance. The quick pulls meant that everyone had to be hyperalert, which drained everyone even further. By the last couple of days, I noticed that all the crew members had a sort of hollow-eyed look. But they never complained, and if I asked Ray or any of the others if they were pushing themselves too hard or needed a rest, the reply was invariably the same: "No, we're fine. Just keep up the strong pulls."

What buoyed all our spirits was the news from the outside. Old friend Andy Roberts was our Mission Control. He was back in Tallahassee, monitoring our progress and serving as a conduit for everyone who wanted to communicate with the guys going where no type 1 diabetics had gone before—or at least not as fast. Andy read or forwarded us e-mails from family and friends, and from sponsors and strangers who were inspired by what we were doing. Almost as important, he kept us in sight of the record and how far ahead of it—and of Beaver Creek—we were. We not only wanted to win, we wanted to be the fastest team ever in RAAM.

Heading into West Virginia, we still had a shot at making that claim, if we could just keep up the intensity. I got a little reckless there. I was going down a mountain, and there was a bend in the road. A sign indicated that the speed limit was thirty miles per hour. As a rule of thumb, if you're on a bike you can usually double the recommended speed of a car on any given stretch of road. That preassumes that the recommended speed is correct. This one apparently wasn't. It should have been fifteen, because suddenly I was making an almost 180-degree turn while going about fifty-five miles per hour. Usually, I love flying downhill on a bike, but when I hit that turn, I knew that I was going way too fast. There was no way I was going to make it; I just had to flatten out the angle so that I didn't crash and really screw up our chances. I went off on this dirt path, hoping that it wouldn't lead me to a precipice. It didn't, but as I turned off the road, my front wheel slipped out, my bike went down, and I rolled into a ditch.

The follow car couldn't see where I'd landed. For all they knew, there had been a cliff there and I was now lying at the bottom of some gorge. But I popped up quickly, jumped out of the ditch and seconds later was back racing down the next mountain. A lot of times, riders become extra-cautious after a crash. My view is, what are the odds I'll crash twice in the same race? And I didn't.

As we approached Atlantic City, we got a new teammate. His name was Josh Kozlowski; he was an eleven-year-old type 1 diabetic from New Jersey who had become one of Team Type 1's biggest fans. Andy had been in touch with Josh's parents, and we arranged to pick him up for the last leg of the race. Josh climbed into the follow car with Ray and the crew and drove the last forty miles to the boardwalk. He was so pumped, so excited to be part of it. "Look at 'em go," Josh exclaimed as he watched Joe, Bob, Nathan, and me speeding toward the finish. "They've got type 1 diabetes like me, and look how fast they go." Even our grizzled crew was moved; I heard later that there wasn't a dry eye in the car.

At the finish line on the boardwalk, Josh was interviewed by local media. "This is *my* team," he said proudly. He was right—Josh and kids like him were a big part of the reason we'd formed Team Type 1. I couldn't have been happier to have had him along for the last part of our adventure. The entire team—Joe, Bub, Nathan, and me, joined by Matt, Bobby, Monique Hanley and Andy Mead—had a police escort as we pedaled down the boardwalk and under the finish banner. We'd done it: we were the first team to finish the 2007 edition of the Race Across America, and we'd done it faster than any other team in the history of the event: 3,046.6 miles in a little over five and half days. A bunch of damn diabetics. How about that? The final results:

Team Type 1: 5 days, 15 hours, 43 minutes (average speed: 22.42 mph)

Beaver Creek-Vail: 5 days, 18 hours, 22 minutes (average speed: 21.99 mph)

We celebrated out there on the boardwalk, the cool Atlantic breezes caressing our sunburned faces. My mom took pictures, Joe's dad told funny stories about bare-assed outdoor showers, and Chris gave me a hug. A TV crew interviewed us, and Josh, and a few people asked for our autographs. After making sure that everything was in order, Ray came ambling over to me. I thought just for once he would break down and give me a hug or tell me something from the heart.

"Phil, I have three words for you and then I need to get some sleep, so you're not going to see me for a while," he said. I leaned forward in anticipation, and he mouthed the words slowly.

"'I . . . hate . . . you.'"

I broke down laughing. Later, I cried—tears of joy and relief—and gave thanks to whatever higher power had put these people in my life. That almost made up for giving me the diabetes.

Forty-eight hours after finishing the Race Across America, I was in a hotel banquet hall in Chicago, talking to five hundred Abbott Pharmaceutical sales reps from around the world. I was there to tell all of them what we'd accomplished and how their technology—the continuous glucose-monitoring system—had helped us to do it. It wasn't baloney, and I wasn't saying this to make them happy. It was true.

I spent the next day in a trade-show booth in Chicago. This was the American Diabetes Association's annual medical conference. There were twelve thousand doctors in attendance—including mine. Nobody had more faith in us than Dr. Bruce Bode, but I think even he was flabbergasted that we'd not only gone the distance but *won,* and in record-setting time.

The only thing that relates to the difficulty of a bike race is a trade show. They're a true grind: days bracketed by meetings at 7:00 A.M. and 10:00 P.M.; talking to people from the breakfast buffet table in the morning, to the bar at night; and standing in a booth, trying to be chipper and enthusiastic, for eight hours in between. Over the course of four days at the convention, I averaged eight hours a day in the booth, two dinners a night, breakfast meetings every morning, and probably two or three other meetings crammed in whenever else I could. I was meeting with sponsors, doctors, sales reps—and, of course, celebrating with my teammates.

For me, the job now became to make Team Type 1 a financially secure, stable, global organization. I didn't want us to be a team of racers that came together once a year for RAAM and then disbanded. I wanted us to become a force in the diabetes community here and abroad. I wanted us to become a professional team.

I wanted to put a Type 1 bike race in the Tour de France by 2012.

This was going to require a different kind of commitment, another level of endurance—and a heckuva lot more sponsorship money.

A week after RAAM, my friends and teammates—the guys with whom I had shared my greatest athletic achievement—were at home, catching up on sleep, getting back to their normal routines, savoring their great achievement. I was still on the road, checking in and out of hotels, making speeches, standing in tradeshow booths, meeting for drinks with potential sponsors; listening and learning; talking, sometimes debating, with doctors and educators and executives about health care, insulin delivery, the type 2 diabetes epidemic, and the latest innovations in diabetes care. This was the beginning of a chaotic new life for me. It started two days after our victory in RAAM, in June 2007, and in many ways it has not stopped since. I did twenty speaking engagements that July alone, attending a seemingly nonstop series of conventions and conferences. My calendar was soon filled with meetings at the headquarters offices of our major sponsors. I began living out of a suitcase; a twenty-five-year-old business traveler, flushed with entrepreneurial enthusiasm and idealism, but increasingly world-weary.

Now, I had two identities: Phil Southerland, the CEO of a fast-growing, not-for-profit organization, and Phil Southerland, the bike racer.

Which Phil would I be, *could* I be? In the flush of our RAAM victory and the heady summer of travel, public speaking, and adulation that followed, I was confident that I could do both, indefinitely. I was wrong, and the resolution of that issue would prove to be painful and sobering.

12

Hop on, Kid

Most RAAM riders will tell you that priority
one is riding your own race,
if you finish 1st or 20th is irrelevant, what is
important is giving it all you got.
—RAAM BLOG 2007

It was the oddest thing. I would be out on a ride, feeling good, but when I picked up the pace, pedaled harder, started to hit the red zone—the point where your body can no longer neutralize lactic acid fast enough, and you begin to fatigue—my left leg would begin to tingle. A few more seconds of hard riding and it would go numb, and I'd feel as if there was no juice, no strength, no life in it at all.

This happened a couple of times in the months leading up to RAAM 2007. But prior to the race, I'd taken ten days off, in part because I was so busy getting things organized that I barely had time to train. Also, I thought some rest before our cross-country ordeal would help. It turned out to be a good move. My legs were fine—or as fine they could be, given what I was asking them to do.

The strange injury, though, returned late in the year. By then I was fully engaged in the growth of our business. But at the same time, I was training, trying to stay sharp for the 2008 season. Joe and I had decided that while Team Type 1 would continue to do RAAM, he and I would now concentrate on developing a professional team, of which we would be a part. We envisioned this team, which would include diabetics and nondiabetic pros, climbing the ranks of professional bike racing to the point that in a few years, we'd be in a position to compete in one of the major European stage races, culminating with the Tour de France.

That was a long-term goal, of course. First off, we had to start making our mark nationally. To that end, we organized a training camp in Buellton, California—an idyllic town in the Santa Ynez Valley, part of California's central coast. A few weeks before camp opened, in January 2008, I went out to nearby Santa Barbara to train with my new pro teammates. Shawn Milne and I were doing a two-mile climb; it was steep and it hurt, as two-mile climbs always will, and we were attacking one another, full gas. We continued neck and neck, attacking and covering each other's moves as we made our way up the mountain. Suddenly, two hundred yards from the top, I felt the telltale tingle in my left leg and . . . *whump.* Almost as if I'd just pulled a power cord out of an outlet. The leg just stopped working. I could barely push the pedal and had to bring the bike to a wobbly stop.

Once I resumed riding at a more comfortable, aerobic pace, feeling came back, and I was fine. It was bizarre—almost as if my leg had a built-in shut-off valve that was triggered whenever I got up to about 85 percent of my maximum intensity. While you might not need to go that hard in recreational cycling, 85 percent intensity and above—the red zone, or "full gas," as we call it—is where a professional bike racer makes his living.

That winter in Buellton, I kept trying to make my living. Every morning at about ten, we'd roll out of the parking lot of Pea Soup Andersen's—a landmark restaurant and hotel that we used as our base. I loved pedaling through the verdant California countryside with Joe, Daniel Holt, and our new pro teammates; I imagined us riding together in the peloton of the big pro races. Some days, it would go well; the leg would feel fine, and I could stay with the leaders. But more often than not, the tingling-numbness-shutdown would kick in whenever I started to push hard. I consulted more physicians, worked with physical therapists, massage therapists, movement therapists . . . you name the therapy, I probably tried it. Nothing helped.

For a while, I tried denial: just pretend it's not a problem, and it will go away. That strategy worked, for a while. In March, Team Type 1 flew to Taiwan, where we finished second overall, and where Shawn became the first Team Type 1 rider to win a stage—a huge achievement for us in a major event.

By spring, I knew I had only one alternative.

On May 5, 2008, I went into the University of Virginia Medical Center, in Charlottesville, for surgery. They were specialists there in this kind of injury, which by now had a name: iliac endofibrosis. The three-hour procedure would involve cutting open three layers of my abdominal muscles, then cutting a ligament that was impinging on the artery and cutting off the blood supply (which explained the numbness). They would then open the iliac artery and clean out scar tissue that had accumulated there. Then, they would do the exact same thing on the femoral artery.

It was the first time in my life I'd been under the knife. Four hours after the procedure, I woke up, itching all over. A doctor gave me a Benadryl, and I fell asleep. A while later, I woke up again—still itching. Another Benadryl and they took me off painkillers. I couldn't get to sleep after that and I was still itchy, and now in pain as well. At 1:00 A.M., I called for a physician. "We're going to give you Benadryl," he said. I was groggy, but not too groggy to get a little annoyed. "It didn't work the first time, it didn't work the second time, so what makes you think it's going to work a third time?" While I respect the training and knowledge of a physician, I'm not afraid to debate or disagree with one, when I think he or she is wrong. And this guy was wrong. Still, you could see that he was not used to being contradicted by a patient. He looked down at me, dumbfounded, and then, said, "Uh . . . Benadryl is the best option . . . er . . . that we have." I looked up at him, straight in the eye, and said, "I'd like another option." He scribbled down something, the nurse gave me something else, and the next day I woke up in great pain but without itchiness.

We clashed also on my diabetes. They wanted to give me a shot of Regular insulin, a slower-acting insulin that I had not used since 1996. I told them that I use a rapid-acting insulin made by Sanofi-Aventis and give myself adjustments on an as-needed basis. It might be five times, might be ten times, it just depends on the situation. They said, "No, this is when you're going to do it." We argued back and forth about the right way to manage my diabetes, a topic about which I consider myself an expert. Finally, I called my endocrinologist, Dr. Bruce Bode, on my cell phone. I handed the phone to the nurse and could hear Bruce's voice booming through the speaker: "Phil is right . . . he needs a rapid insulin, on an as-needed basis. Listen to him, he's the world's number-one diabetic!"

I had to stifle a laugh as I nodded firmly in agreement. *There's my next T-shirt,* I thought. *"World's #1 Diabetic." Has a nice ring to it.*

Still, being a "prominent" diabetic had its drawbacks. Eleven days after the surgery on my leg, I was at another diabetes conference. I didn't want to go, I probably shouldn't have gone, but the sponsors pleaded with me. I was still supposed to be off my feet at this point; the farthest I'd walked was down the block to the local Starbucks from my house in Atlanta, and that had felt like a fifty-mile ride. So, standing and walking around for eight hours on the trade-show floor in Orlando was definitely not what the doctor had ordered. In order to keep the pain at bay, I popped Vicodin like Junior Mints. After a while, it didn't matter. Behind forced smiles and pleasantries with sponsors and endocrinologists, I was in agony. It was a jarring reminder that my two roles in Team Type 1—owner and rider—were becoming incompatible. Doubts began to cloud my mind as to whether I really could continue to race for the team while trying to manage and grow the business at the same time.

Rehab from my surgery was very tricky. I had been told that if my blood pressure increased too much in the arteries, the patches could pop, and—as we were dealing with two large arteries—I could die. Needless to say, that got my attention. I was able to tamp down my usual instincts to do as much training as I could, as fast as I could. Instead, I followed the script: three weeks after surgery, I was allowed to begin gentle aquatic exercise. I went to the local pool, found a lane, and paddled back and forth on a kickboard for twenty minutes. To me, there's nothing more boring than doing laps in a pool. It was especially bad when senior citizens, little kids, and overweight people went chugging past me. To think that a hotshot young bike racer should come to this! It was demoralizing.

A few weeks later, I was on an exercise bike, which I hate almost as much as the pool. Most of my riding colleagues would agree with me there—when you're a road cyclist, used to the excitement and stimuli of the outdoors, pedaling nowhere fast seems like someone's sadistic vision of hell.

Still, I knew it was prudent and necessary to get me back to where I wanted to be. On June 27, 2008—about eight weeks after the surgery—I climbed back on my bike for the first time. I pedaled around my neighborhood for an hour and was exhausted. Over the course of that summer, I gradually built up to two hours, three hours. For the first six weeks, I was keeping my heart rate low—applying less force to the pedals, making sure the intensity level was low. In late summer, I began picking it up. In October, I did my first bike race in nearly half a year. I was rounding back into shape, and just in time. In February, I would be competing in the most prestigious race of my career. Team Type 1 had been invited to participate in the Tour of California.

Tour of California
Stage 1: Sunday, February 15
Davis–Santa Rosa
107.6 miles

A few minutes before noon on Sunday, February 15, I sat nervously in a pack of one hundred bike racers in the middle of downtown Davis, California.

This was the first stage of the 2009 Amgen Tour of California, and considering the severity of my surgery, I knew that it was a small miracle that I was there at all. The 2009 race boasted the most impressive cast of professional bike racers ever to drop wheels on American asphalt: Levi Leipheimer, Tom Boonen, Fabian Cancellara, Fränk and Andy Schleck, Jens Voigt, Mark Cavendish, and George Hincapie competed, not to mention a rider who had come out of retirement for this season—a fellow named Lance.

That year, Lance Armstrong rode for Astana in a support role for his American teammate Leipheimer, the two-time defending champ of the Tour of California. There were sixteen other teams competing against them, including the big-team names of bike racing such as Columbia-High Road, Saxo Bank, Rabobank, and

Garmin-Slipstream—plus a new name on the tour roster, Team Type 1.

As I looked around me, seeing the guys I'd idolized and whose careers I'd followed for years, I thought about my own road to this point. Since the surgery, I had done everything possible to get myself prepared for this day. I was on a strict diet, training hard, doing my rehab. Wouldn't you know it, though, my diabetes—usually in control—had decided to throw me a curveball in the last month leading up to the tour. For some reason, my blood sugar had been going up at night. I'd go to bed with a perfect reading and wake up with a blood sugar of 180. That shouldn't be happening in your sleep. I consulted with Howard Zisser, an endocrinologist I'd met at a conference. Dr. Zisser was with the Sansum Diabetes Research Institute in Santa Barbara. (Sansum is an important name in the history of diabetes treatment: in 1922, the founder of the institute, Dr. William Sansum, became the first physician in the United States to produce and administer insulin to patients with diabetes.)

Dr. Zisser and I brainstormed some possible solutions. As usual when dealing with my diabetes, we were often in uncharted territory. Few people with type 1 have participated in endurance athletic events of the level of duration and intensity that I was trying to do. Finally, we came up with a strategy that worked: I started taking my basal insulin and then an injection of rapid-acting insulin before bed. This was totally different from anything I'd ever done before, and got the blood sugar back under control. We never did figure out why that overnight spike had occurred; perhaps it was a reminder that sometimes, diabetes management is an ongoing experiment. No matter how perfect the system, how good the technology, your disease can sometimes take an unpredictable turn. The way to handle it? Don't panic. If you can't figure out a reason, don't worry, just figure out a solution. Which is what I did, with the help of Dr. Zisser.

Now I had only to figure out how to compete in a stage race with the world's best bike racers. Matt Wilson, one of our new Team Type 1 pros, was really helpful. An Australian, Matt was a veteran of years of competition in Europe. Like a lot of the pros we signed, he was impressed by the team's mission, even though he was not himself a diabetic. Let's be honest: he was also impressed with our sponsorship. In the bike-racing world, teams come and go, as their sponsors change or, in some cases, go out of business. Most of our riders know that companies like Sanofi-Aventis and Abbott are not likely to go out of business.

Matt was a survivor—he'd finished 141st in the Tour de France. I, on the other hand, would have been lucky to finish 141st in the Tour of California—even though there were only 136 riders in the race. At this point in my career, and especially with my leg injury, I realized my limits; I knew where I stood in the hierarchy of professional cyclists. Matt was my type of bike racer: he knew how to work hard, to make the most out of the talent he had; he knew how to look at stage profiles, knew the best way to help his team. Before the race, he patiently gave me some tips on how I could do the same.

The wind was blowing hard through downtown Davis at the start. If the big guns of the Tour of Cali decided to make it hard, it was going to be difficult for those of us hanging on the back. But just five miles into the race, Francisco Mancebo, of Rock Racing, along with my buddy Tim Johnson, of Team OUCH, broke away, and the group of sprinters was off and running (he would maintain that lead and end up winning the stage). An early breakaway was perfect for me: it meant that the overall pace of the peloton would be a bit slower. So I was able to get on Matt's wheel and stay with the pack. As the 107-mile stage wore on, the rain got steadier. It was cold, and I kept eating because I knew my blood sugar would drop. When we hit a short, steep climb, I used Matt's suggestion of asking the crowd to give me a hand—literally. I got pushes and shoves from the rain-gear-clad spectators gathered along the road. Late in the stage, the pace picked up, and I started to drop back. In the last few kilometers, it was me and another new Type 1 teammate, Fabio Calabria, a talented young Australian rider who *was a* diabetic, like me. Fabio and I rode together through the end of that stage, in Santa Rosa. The important thing was that we finished—and made the cutoff time. That was the goal for the day. It was the first time that two diabetics had competed in a major stage race of this caliber—and probably one of the few times that two diabetics competed together in any major professional sports event.

Stage 2: Monday, February 16
Sausalito–Santa Cruz
115.9 miles

February 16, 2009 was a big day for the Tour of California, as we would have the honor of riding ceremoniously across the Golden Gate Bridge—one of the first times the bridge was closed for an event.

The bridge was a neutral zone, meaning that we simply rode over it as a group. Still, while we were not yet racing, we were all on our toes. Unfortunately, the weather didn't cooperate—again, it was raining and cold, around forty degrees—and the metal plates of the bridge were slick with rain. We had to pay full attention to avoid crashing. I couldn't stop and look out over the Bay and admire or appreciate the significance of the moment—but in retrospect, it was a privilege to be part of such a special moment in the history of American cycling.

As soon as we were off the bridge, the race started—and started fast. We were flying, and I was dying. Still, I pedaled furiously to stay with the peloton through the first climb. If I was dropped this early, I knew, I'd be finished.

There were moments early in this stage when I wanted to quit. It would have been so much easier. I began talking to myself, repeating a mantra I sometimes used when the going got really bad in a race: "pain is temporary, success is forever, pain is temporary, success is forever. . . ." Sounds like the kind of cliché you'd see stenciled on the wall of a high school gym, but hey, it works. Mercifully, the pack slowed down, and I got back into the thick of things. At about forty miles, we hit this climb at a place called Bonny Doon Road. I ended up in a group of fifteen guys, including some big names, such as Fred Rodriguez and Francesco Chicci—both stage winners at the Giro d'Italia. But neither of them was a climber. Up and down we went, riding along the Northern California coast, the rain pelting us. Now my focus was again on making the cutoff time, which is calculated as a percentage of the winner's time.

I knew it was 7 percent, but not everybody else did. When Rodriguez asked what the cutoff time was and I told him, there were a few seconds of silence as fifteen riders did the math in their heads. Let's see . . . we were forty kilometers and fourteen minutes behind the leaders, who would finish in about five hours, or three hundred minutes; 7 percent of that is twenty-one. Twenty-one minutes! That's all the time we had to finish. Our pack reacted as if someone had stuck firecrackers in our butts. We took off, determined to make the cutoff. Without any communication, we began to rotate the lead. We knew that was the way to do it. One guy went to the head of the pack and pulled for ten seconds, then got off. Another guy took his place. So, like a giant rotating wheel of bike racers, working together, we made our way along the road to Santa Cruz.

One of the guys with us was Brad Huff, a sprinter for the Jelly Belly team. As we all rode toward the finish, he came up to me. "Man, you guys on Team Type 1 are awesome," he said. I thanked him. He then called out to the other riders. "Hey guys," he said to the rest of the pack, pointing to Fabio and me, "these two are rock stars. They are saving lives!"

Maybe so, but we weren't doing much to save our time. We appreciated the love we got from a lot of the riders at the tour, but we really wanted to be taken seriously as a pro racing team, not as a "bunch of diabetics." While Fabio and I made the cutoff, one of our climbers dropped out of the race; the other guys were not riding as well as they had hoped, and my mood was pretty low that night—until I got on my laptop to write one of my Tour blog posts that we were posting on the Team Type 1 Web site. When I logged on, I saw forty-eight personal messages. They were from people I knew and total strangers. But all of them were expressing encouragement, telling me how inspired they were, how great it was what we were doing, how their kids were following along. It was just like RAAM. I remembered then that while we did indeed want to earn respect as a pro team, my real goal here was something else: it was part of my mission to help inspire and galvanize the diabetes community. Every day I stayed in the race would help further that goal.

Stage 3: Tuesday, February 17
San Jose–Modesto
Miles: 104.2

Day three, and I had two new problems: first, tendinitis in my left ankle, which made it painful to stroke the pedals. Second, a four-mile climb, with an average grade of 10 percent. And of course, these were added to my ongoing problems—bad weather, the fear of my leg going dead, not to mention a whacky metabolism, my blood sugar undulating like the coastal hills we were riding.

The climb at Sierra Road happened early, only ten kilometers in the stage, and it was full gas all the way. My left leg started hurting. I had to pull up to the team car, and while I held on to the roof, our team physician cut the tape off my ankle to relieve some of the pressure. Shortly afterward, another issue: I could feel my Navigator vibrating, alerting me that my blood sugar was either too high or too low. The problem was that I couldn't tell, because my gloves were so thick and my hands so numb that I couldn't pull the Navigator out of my pocket. Again, I waved the car up to me; the doc reached out the window, grabbed my jersey, and pulled out the Navigator. It showed that my blood pressure was 133 and going straight down. He gave me a Coke, some gels, and again, I rejoined the race.

For about forty miles, I was alone as I raced to catch up to the peloton. I finally reached the follow vehicles, so I knew I was close. As I'm navigating through slow-moving cars, I look to my left— there's Lance Armstrong on the side of the road, stretching his quads. If I was anywhere near Lance in this race, I knew I was okay. I continued along and soon passed three of his Astana teammates who had hung back waiting for the Boss (actually, Levi Leipheimer was the Astana star that year, and he would eventually win the race, but of course, Lance is . . . well, *Lance*. So he gets the star treatment no matter what his role in a race).

A few minutes later, I looked back and here come those three Astana riders with Lance on their wheel. He turned to me and smiled. "Hop on, kid!" he said. I got on his wheel and it was a free ride back to the peloton. So, for one glorious moment, I followed Lance Armstrong to the front of the pack.

At the end of the stage, I was relieved to have survived another day. Others hadn't: by now only 119 riders remained of the original 136. Our team lost another key guy that day, as Ian McGregor crashed and had to quit. I finished 113th—five seconds behind Carlos Sister, the winner of the 2008 Tour de France. I kind of felt bad for him, being back there with us slugs, so I let him finish 112th.

Stage 4: Wednesday, February 18
Merced–Clovis
Miles: 115.4

Finally, some warm California sunshine! And flat terrain for the first fifty kilometers. The pack was in the mood to race that day. I wanted so much to be part of that race, of this tour, but suddenly it all came apart. I had no power on my left side. My ankle ached and my quadriceps went numb. It was as if my body were just shutting down. When we were about to hit the mountainous part of the stage, I finally pulled the plug. I had done the calculations in my head, and I knew there was no way I was going to make the cut-off. I waved down the car. "I'm done," I said, and climbed in. We drove on the road a few clicks, and there was Fabio by the side of the road. He got in the car, too. When you pull out of a stage race, it's a depressing experience, so there was no talking in the team car. When I got to my hotel room later, I collapsed and tried to put it all in perspective. Yeah, I'd had to quit, and that left a bad taste. Still, I thought, we'd made it through half the tour, and gone where no diabetics had gone before.

We had three riders left, all nondiabetics. We were there for them in Escondido a few days later, cheering on our three teammates as they finished the Tour of California. We were fourteenth out of sixteen in the team category—a bad day for Team Type 1.

Our next event was the Tour of Taiwan, a major event on the other side of the world. I was still not willing to accept my leg injury, and kept training. At first, I thought maybe somehow I'd beaten it. We got to Taiwan, and I started out the race flying. I felt great—until I crashed a quarter of the way through the stage. The second day: someone takes me out again. This was spooky: it's rare that any rider endures two crashes in a row. The third day, I get to a climb, and my leg dies. Just dies. Clearly, whatever they'd done in the surgery was not working; a major operation, six weeks of recovery, and weeks and months of rehab—all for nothing. I spent about three hours by myself that day, walking around this little town in Taiwan, looking deep inside myself. Was I really meant to be a pro bike racer? Did I want to remain in the sport as an owner, even if I couldn't compete? Should I abandon Team Type 1 and try to help diabetics in another way? Or maybe I should just say screw it all and go back to selling insurance. Maybe the epiphany I'd had when I helped Joe Eldridge change his lifestyle had run its course. That was almost five years in the past. We'd accomplished a lot, done a lot, helped many diabetics. Now maybe it was somebody else's turn.

I flew home and didn't ride for ten days. Then, as had happened before, I got back on the bike and was able to ride; the strength I'd built up from Cali and Taiwan enable me to ride despite the numbness. I took second in a regional race, helped Joe win another. This was a glimmer of hope. Could I go back to competitive riding? I tried to make it work at the race I knew best. At the Twilight Criterium in Athens in April 2009, I dropped out after sixteen laps, with a leg that felt like someone was choking it.

Now, I went to a vascular surgeon in Atlanta. He tested me on a stationary bike while measuring blood pressure and flow into my leg. Then they did an MRI of the artery. The results: I was getting only about two-thirds of the blood to my left leg that I should have when I biked at higher intensity. "I'm sorry," said the surgeon when we met to discuss the results. "The problem has returned. And it appears to be even worse than it was. There's really nothing we can do now. Surgery at this point won't do a thing." That was it. You can't function as a bike racer when your leg is getting only two-thirds of the blood it is supposed to. You might as well try to race at Daytona with a car that has a deflated tire, or a clogged fuel line. It's just not going to work. My professional racing career was over. Depression set in, but I soon found what I thought was a surefire way to deal with it.

13

The Italian Job

I think it's fair to say that *'l Tour e' piu grande, ma che il Giro e' piu bello.'* That the Tour is bigger but that now the Giro d'Italia is more beautiful. I like that comparison.

—ANGELO ZOMEGNAN, DIRECTOR, GIRO D'ITALIA, QUOTED ON *CyclingNews.com*, MAY 2010

"Hello?" said the voice on the line.

I paused for a moment before responding. This had been a difficult call to make, but one I knew I had to, because I'd finally admitted to myself that I was in trouble.

"Hi, Dad," I said. "It's me."

It was June 2009—two months after Twilight, and a few weeks after I'd sat in my spandex Team Type 1 bike racing clothes, feeling like an impostor, at the satellite media tour in New York City. Shortly after that, another type 1 team had won RAAM, setting another record. This was our third time winning the eight-person-team division, and the third time the team had set a record. But I wasn't a part of it. Joe and I had stopped racing RAAM after 2007 and let others take our place. We figured there was plenty of glory left for us, racing as part of the type 1 professional team that we had launched with much fanfare in January 2008.

For Joe, the plan seemed to be working perfectly. He had only gotten stronger since the days of our burrito bets. When we first met, I was by far the better cyclist. That changed pretty quickly. Joe is now lean, powerful, confident. He's gotten to be a great sprinter, and he's an integral part of our lead-out train for the finish, meaning that he gets our sprinters into perfect finishing position in our big races. Seven years earlier, he was getting his ass kicked in beginners' races. Cycling is a long, slow grind to the top and Joe was diligent in his work. In the last seven years, he's lost about forty-five pounds. He looks like a bike racer now, not like a linebacker who decided to go for a bike ride.

I'm proud of how far he's come.

For me, dropping out of the Tour of California in February 2009 had been hard—but at least I'd been able to finish three stages of the most prestigious grand tour in the United States. The crashes in Taiwan, the results of the test on my artery, and my embarrassing finish at Twilight in April 2009—a race I probably should never even have started—well, that was like three trucks in a row running over an already dented frame. There was no denying it now: I could no longer race; I could barely ride.

Suddenly, the thing I loved to do best in life was unavailable. Bicycling was more than competition for me: it was a lifestyle, a culture, and it was also a form of medicine as effective as the insulin I took for diabetes. As anyone who walks even thirty minutes a day will tell you, regular physical activity has a profound effect on your psyche. My hours of training did more than keep me lean; they kept me sane. Now it was gone, I thought, and yet I still had all the pressures and responsibilities of before. Not to mention the constant job of managing my disease.

In the weeks after Twilight, I had started doing two things, one of them good, the other not so much.

Needing an athletic goal, as well as something to keep me fit, I had started to run a couple of miles a day. It wasn't like cycling— I couldn't go for nearly as long, far, or fast in a pair of Nikes as I could on my Orbea. Still, it helped me break a sweat, it was a challenge. To give my running some focus, rather than just plod along a few miles every day, I had also shaped a goal: I would run the 2009 New York City Marathon, and break three hours—hardly an Olympic performance, but a time that was out of the grasp of the vast majority of the nearly forty thousand people who did that race. I entered the lottery and was accepted for the race, held the first Sunday in November.

That was good.

The nightly bouts of drinking that followed my running—that accompanied most of my business meetings, not to mention my social engagements—were not so good. Not so good at all.

Part of this was simply a bad attitude. At that point, I had come to hate my bike; as if it was the bicycle and not my leg that had betrayed me. I was also sick of hearing people asking me about it. "How's the biking?" "How's your racing?" I got tired of having to explain the injury, the surgery—and decided I liked the feeling of being buzzed on a few drinks a lot better.

Part of this was a product of my lifestyle. The treadmill that I had seemingly and unknowingly stepped on after our victory in RAAM 2007 had never really stopped. It had whisked me, seemingly in the blink of an eye, from city to city, corporate headquarters to trade-show booth to conference suite to medical center corner office. These had been punctuated by training camps and bike races here and overseas, but now that I was more of a team official than a team rider, my role in the building of the business of Team Type 1 was the top priority.

As any frequent business traveler can tell you, a life spent "up in the air" is rife with temptation and opportunity to drink. I was doing that with an alarming frequency. Yet, like many, I managed to rationalize the vodka tonics I was knocking down with clients and sponsors: having a drink was part of doing business, I told myself, and if I was going to drink, then this was perfect, because tonic raised my blood sugar, vodka lowered it. *Hey,* I tried to convince myself, *drinking is practically medicinal.*

This was, of course, an utter self-deception, and the two drinks had become four and five; the libations seemed to start earlier and earlier, the fuzzy-headed mornings more frequent. Still, I argued to myself, this was part of the price of doing business.

Who was I kidding? Now I sometimes felt that I had no home. I traveled constantly. In 2008, I was on the road 197 days. At this point, halfway through 2009, I was on track to 240.

I was drinking too much and too often. The night prior to making the call to my father, I had spent time visiting children at a local hospital in Long Beach, California. Then I got trashed that night at a local bar. So now, with guilt and a crushing hangover, I was driving back to my hotel after lunch. Later I'd be headed to LAX for a flight home to Atlanta, and in the back of my mind I was already looking forward to drinks in the airport lounge, drinks on the plane. No good. I knew the call I had to make.

"How are you, Dad?"

"Doing well, son. It's always good to hear from you."

I knew that for most of my life I wouldn't have been able to say the same about him. For years we'd been estranged. There was a period of my life, from about the ages of twelve to eighteen, where it was maybe once a year; a birthday card, a phone call that I usually terminated quickly. I still burned with resentment at what I felt was his awful behavior toward Joanna and me during their divorce. I had a certain expectation of what a father should be and do, and how he ought to have made a greater effort to be a part of his son's life . . . even when the son was no longer under his roof. In his absence, I had spent much of my life gravitating toward substitutes, whether it was a "nearby guy" like Kevin Davis, a group of surrogate big brothers like the Revolutions boys, or an avuncular figure like David Crowe. Not surprisingly, my father didn't see it that way, and felt that I had continually rebuffed his efforts to restore our relationship. Again, there was probably some truth there, as well.

In recent years we had begun to converse occasionally. It was usually small talk, but not this time.

"Dad, I need to talk to you about something." I fumbled with the words, trying to figure out how to broach this topic. "You know, I fly first class a lot and the first thing they do up there is offer you a drink. . . . I'm out all the time, in social situations, as part of my business . . . and . . . uh . . ."

"Yes?"

"Well, I guess what I'm trying to say is that it's about the drinking. When does doing it 'some' turn into doing it too much, turn into 'having a problem'?"

My dad, who had retired from Florida State University in 2008, had been in AA since 1983, and to his credit had not taken a drink since the day Joanna had called him from my grandparents' house and delivered her ultimatum. But the buildup to that point had been a long one.

"My own history was not one of sudden alcoholism, but rather a very gradual increase over the years," he explained, in the erudite manner that reminded me, every time I talked to him, that this was a man who had lectured on the law for three decades. He told me that his drinking had started with a glass of brandy or scotch when he came home. One had turned to two and three, and eventually it was taking over his life. I'd never heard any of this and was fascinated. But then he turned it back to my situation.

"If you get to the point where the most important part of your day is the drinking, then you know you've got issues," Dad said.

It was a brief but helpful conversation. I knew what I needed to do, what I needed to watch for. I'd be lying if I said I haven't imbibed since I talked to him in June 2009, but my drinking has definitely decreased; there have been weeks when I've gone without it entirely, and when I say I'm having only "one or two," it really is one or two. That said, I realize that the urge to drink excessively is something I'm always going to have to be on guard against.

Dad later said he wasn't shocked by the call. "It came as no surprise, because alcoholism is a genetic disease," he said. "It runs in my family, so I would not be surprised if Phil had had to do a little experimentation."

The discussions between my dad and me have moved on to other things, although we have tried not to reopen old wounds. What's done is done. I also know that there are two sides to every story. The side you're hearing is mine and Joanna's. I don't know where our relationship will go in the future, but at least we finally have a relationship.

At least and at last, I have a father, again.

Much of the period from early May through mid-June 2009—the weeks after the Twilight Criterium—was a blur: I probably accumulated about fifteen thousand frequent flyer miles, spent maybe a total of ten days at home in Atlanta, and shook more hands than a candidate for Congress. There were sponsor meetings, conventions, and trade shows to attend. There were races across the country in which Team Type 1 was competing—a total of twenty days that month alone—and even though I couldn't ride with them, I still had to be on hand for every race; to meet race organizers, strategize with sponsors, make sure that all my riders were happy campers, sign checks, and help provide the public face and voice of our team and our mission.

No matter where I was, there were still the regular conference calls and the late-night e-mail exchanges with athletes and agents on the other side of the world, not to mention the personal messages we get from parents of kids with diabetes, looking for advice or encouragement. I also had to make sure that fifty-six bike riders were paid and that they and their agents were happy. I had a staff to look after. I was on the phone with Vassili and our other team director, Gord Fraser; I had to negotiate a contract with one rider, try to hire another, and consider whether a third was going to work out for us long term. There were photo shoots, a Web site upgrade to oversee, interviews with reporters; and there were the kinds of things that all business owners must deal with—meetings with lawyers and accountants on things routine, productive, and occasionally headache inducing.

As far as my new athletic goal, I never did run the 2009 New York City Marathon—although I still may run the race somewhere down the road. To add injury to injury, I started feeling pain in my leg while running that summer. I thought it was related to the arterial problem, but my doctor suggested an MRI, which revealed a stress fracture. I'd done too much too soon. No marathon, no running for a while.

However, the month that I would have been running in New York, I was invited to ride in El Tour de Tucson, one of the largest open-participant events in the country. Many of the eight thousand riders do so to raise funds for various charities. I came out to Tucson for El Tour to speak to the ninety-five riders who were raising funds for the Juvenile Diabetes Research Foundation. Being with them, and then riding as part of this event, was energizing, inspiring—and best of all, pain-free. My leg didn't seize up, nor did it in the six months since, allowing me to train regularly again (including with many of my old Tallahassee buddies, when I'm down there visiting my mom).

Although I probably will never again be able to compete at the level I once did, I can still ride a bike. For that I am grateful. I should also add that I am breathing, upright, and fully able to read the eye chart in my doctor's office—all things that Joanna was told would be unlikely prospects for me by the time I reached twenty-five.

What motivates me today is not the chance of winning a bike race but of changing behaviors on a national scale. The Centers for Disease Control estimates that one out of every three children born in the United States since 2000 will become a type 2 diabetic. That's a horrifying statistic, and it compelled me to expand Team Type 1's mission beyond those with the form of diabetes that I have—which is not preventable—to type 2, which is. Part of that prevention involves better nutrition and more physical activity, which is where our team of riders can provide some good role models for these kids.

That team has expanded in the last year: currently, we have a total of 101 riders on seven different teams. They are male, female, younger, older, professional, amateur, people with type 1 and type 2 diabetes. We now have twenty-five full-time paid staff, as well.

Even more important, Team Type 1 has become involved in diabetes care on a global level. We've recently formed a partnership with the International Diabetes Federation. We're working on their Life for a Child program, the goal of which is to provide basic care for juvenile diabetics the world over. Our goal is to provide insulin, blood sugar meters, and test strips to the seventy-four thousand children with type 1 who are not getting insulin on a regular basis. We're on our way to meeting that goal.

Not bad for an organization that began as a vague idea in the overexercised mind of a twenty-two-year-old during a crazy, three-hundred-mile ride home.

What's it like to be the owner of a professional bike-racing team? You might think the job sounds glamorous—flying first class to exotic places, hanging out with the top names in the sport, sipping expensive drinks with sponsors and agents at luxury European resort hotels and restaurants.

The truth is, while there might be a little of that, there's a lot more of this: hard work, intense preparation, occasional rejection, and, even when you get a "yes," huge pressure to deliver on what you have promised, while ensuring that whatever the "yes" was for, it's going to help your team grow, as well.

The challenge is particularly great for us. We're a relatively small American racing team—we're not Columbia, Garmin, Rabobank, or one of the other big, established outfits—and our mission is different from any other team's. That challenge becomes even more onerous when you're dealing with the biggest events in the sport.

Such is the case with the Giro d'Italia.

Going into the spring of 2010, I knew that in order for Team Type 1 to continue to expand, we had to start competing in bigger and more prestigious races. And there are very, very few more prestigious than the Giro, generally regarded as the second-most-important grand tour, behind only the Tour de France. Name a top rider, a top team from any era, and chances are they've competed in the Giro, whose century-old pedigree is nearly equal to that of Le Tour.

Our entrée to the Giro came through our coach Vassili, who had competed in Italy as a rider and is still as respected in the cycling world there as he is on our team. "Pheel," said Vassili. "You must meet Angelo. Very smart . . . he will understand what Team Type 1 is all about. Angelo is the man. He *is* the Giro."

Through Vassili, and another sponsor of ours, I was able to arrange a meeting with Angelo Zomegnan, director of the Giro and one of the sport's great impresarios.

A former journalist, Zomegnan moved into cycling management, took over directorship of the Giro, and has made a great event even better. He does it with panache, too, and sometimes with ideas that leave traditionalists in the cycling world shaking their fists with outrage (such as his plan to hold a stage of the Giro in Washington, D.C., in 2012). *The New York Times* called him "a maestro of marketing," which was music to my ears. I admired Angelo and his approach to the sport. There is a rich tradition in bike racing, yes, and that's a beautiful part of the sport, but there's nothing wrong with change, either. Angelo seemed like an innovator; maybe, I thought, he would be the kind of man who could understand what a team like ours brought to the table. A team designed not just to win stages or jerseys but to spread a message of hope to millions of people afflicted with a disease.

In late April 2010, we were able to arrange a meeting with Angelo as his office in Milan. He arrived, impeccably dressed as he always is, in a stylish suit. He was polite but businesslike, just as I'd expected. I hoped he saw a little of the same in the fellow on the opposite side of the conference table. One of my concerns is that now, as a twenty-eight-year-old who still looks about twenty-two, I'm not going to be taken seriously in the halls of power, especially European power. From what I'd heard about Angelo, I figured he wasn't overly concerned about that. My feeling was that if he perceived what we had to offer as something fresh and new and that could help his race, he probably wouldn't have cared if I was wearing diapers.

My real concern was the language. While I was confident that I could sell the unique qualities of Team Type 1, I'd never had to do it through an interpreter.

So when Angelo, sat down, offered his hand, and said, "Hello, Phil, nice to meet you," I was relieved. "Ah, English," I said, grinning. Angelo smiled back and waved his hand. "No problem," he said, and sat back to listen to my pitch.

I told him, in a very condensed form, my story—the one you've read in this book. I told him about where I came from and where I was going. I told him a little about the who and the what of Team Type 1 and a lot more about the why. And as I explained to him what we were trying to do—about our efforts to help Third World kids get the test strips and insulin they so desperately need; our hopes to help find a cure for diabetes; about our close partnerships not only with the pharmaceuticals but with the medical community and the research institutions and public health agencies in the United States and elsewhere—I saw Angelo's gaze rise up and over me. He had been listening intently and now seemed focused on something located just above my right shoulder. For a second I thought, *Am I boring him to death?* But no, I had been in enough meetings to know the look of someone who has been struck by a good idea. I realized that my message had resonated. He *got* it. He understood what we were trying to do, and its importance, and was now thinking about exactly how it could benefit the Giro.

I'd like to tell you that I walked out of there with a signed contract. But that's not the way it works in this business. What I got from Angelo, actually, was something even better.

A challenge.

"If you want to be in my race, Phil," he said, after I'd finished my pitch, "we need a good biological passport for all your riders." Instituted by the UCI, the professional cyclists' union, in 2008, this is a digital record of each rider, in which the results of all doping tests over a period of time are collated. It's the latest and, the UCI believes, most effective way to find the cheaters who've been a plague on our sport.

Second, Angelo said, "You must have the right DNA." At first, I thought this also had something to do with profiling for banned substances, but Angelo explained: "By that, I mean the right chemistry of riders. The Giro, we are known for exciting races. I want a team who will give us that. Excitement." I understood. Good cause or not, it made no sense for him to bring a team of eight guys who would struggle at the back of the pack. He wasn't expecting us necessarily to challenge the powerhouse teams, but he was expecting us to be competitive. That meant we needed to show up with a good sprinter, climber, time trialist—maybe a guy who had a shot of finishing in the top ten overall. Not to mention some riders who would take risks, who wouldn't hesitate to jump into a breakaway.

We had guys like this—and I knew we'd be able to recruit a couple more. Not household names, but gutsy, talented riders; riders who had helped Team Type 1's pro team to stage wins and podium spots at the tours of Ireland, Mexico, California, and other competitive races. Guys like Rubens Bertogilati, Alexander Efim-kin, and Javier Megias Leal—a twenty-seven-year-old type 1 diabetic from Madrid. *Boy,* I thought, *would I love to see Javier crossing the line in a sprint at the Giro.*

"I know we can do that, Mr. Zomegnan," I said. "We will deliver good DNA."

He smiled.

"Okay, Phil, last thing."

"What's that?"

"We must get to know each other," he said. "I must know who you are, the program you're trying to build." Meet these three challenges successfully, he said in conclusion, "Maybe there's a chance you can do our race."

I left the meeting walking on air. I've loved a challenge ever since I was riding in Tallahassee with the Revolutions crew—and if the challenge now didn't involve my racing, it did involve my racing team. In the next few weeks, we gathered together more-detailed information about our team, our program, our riders. We began to negotiate with some new riders. We sent Angelo and his people more-detailed and comprehensive reports on who we were, what we'd done, and what we could do.

I also accepted his invitation to come over and watch the Giro in May 2010. He was busy, of course, so I didn't get to see much of him, but I did get to watch one of the most exciting bike races I'd ever seen, not to mention one of the great sports spectacles. This year, it started hundreds of miles away, in Amsterdam (more hand-wringing from the purists), then picked up in Italy, through magnificent countryside and awe-inspiring mountains (some cycling aficionados think the scenery in the Giro is even more beautiful than in the Tour de France, which is saying something). The great

Italian rider Ivan Basso won the race, but the Australians did very well, too—a point that Angelo made in some of the postrace interviews I heard. He recognizes the importance of bringing more of the English-speaking world—fans as well as riders—into his event. I particularly appreciated what he told a reporter from *Cycling News*. "We've only just started on a long road of change and innovation that will be good for cycling and especially good for the Giro," he reportedly said. "Some people think we're pushing things too far, making too many changes, making the racing too hard. But I don't think change is a problem. I think it's a good thing. Perhaps, we're changing things a little too fast but better too much than too little."

Since the appearance in the 2011 race of a team founded by a diabetic from Tallahassee, Florida, would most definitely be counted under the category of "change" in the 102-year-old Giro, this was music to my ears. Meanwhile, I was beginning to make some changes of my own. I was reorienting much of my business across the Atlantic. This, I began to realize, was where our future lay. Even though the sport has increased dramatically in popularity in the United States, we all know that Europe is the epicenter of bike racing. I make the analogy to basketball in China. It's a huge sport there, and they've contributed a couple of superstars to the game. But, much as they love hoops in China, it's still an American game, and the best teams and players are found here. Same with bike racing—the United States may be the largest potential market, and certainly we've had some great American riders in the last few years, starting with Lance. But I think even he would agree that bike racing's "home field" is and probably always will be Europe.

To that end, Team Type 1 opened an office in Tuscany—not for from Angelo's office in Milan—in November 2011. Also, as part of my new transatlantic strategy, I started taking Italian and French lessons, so that I could raise my game to the level where people like Angelo were playing—multilingual, international, smart, and successful.

And also, because I thought it would be a sign of respect.

In July, more news: I was invited to attend the Tour de France. I arrived for the last few days, in time to watch Alberto Contador and Andy Schleck battle it out. The night after the last stage, I met Angelo for dinner. We were in a bistro in Paris, with a view of the Eiffel Tower behind us—where just a few hours before, a victorious Contador and his team had come streaming triumphantly down the Champs-Elysées.

I tried a little of my Italian on him, and he smiled. "Not bad," Angelo said.

We spoke in English about the business, about the team, about his event. It was, as they say, a wide-ranging discussion. After we had finished nibbling on *le fromage*—the traditional board of cheese served at the end of a dinner in France—he looked at me and cleared his throat. "I am impressed with what you have done so far," he said, "and how seriously you have worked to meet the conditions I set out only three months ago."

"Thank you," I said.

"Phil," he continued, "I think your team will help a lot of people around the world. And through my race, we can impact many lives. I want to invite Team Type 1 to the 2011 Giro."

I really don't remember all that much of the rest of that evening—except that I had a date with a lovely young lady, who probably got very bored with me, glassy-eyed, going on and on about Angelo and the Giro.

I couldn't help it: this was a red-letter day for Team Type 1.

And so, on May 8, 2011, Team Type 1—a squad that will likely include several type 1 diabetics—will ride in the Giro d'Italia, alongside Tour de France and former Giro champ Contador as well as defending champ Basso, former Tour winner Carlos Sister, Cadel Evans, Alexander Vinokourov, and Christian Vande Velde.

A few weeks later, we got the word that the management of the Tour de France was interested in hearing our proposal for Team Type 1's participation in their fabled event, perhaps as early as 2012. The Giro and the Tour have a close relationship and one of mutual respect. Christian Prudhome, the director of the Tour, and Angelo are good friends. I don't know if he put in a good word for us, but if he did, I am grateful.

The Giro. Le Tour. It's the dream of every bike racer to compete in races like these. I once had that dream, too. And as I write this, in November 2010, it looks like it's going to come true. Only not quite in the way I expected it. Just the same, it's still a sweet, sweet feeling.

After my last European trip, I hopped on my bike and pedaled off into the Georgia countryside. I still can't race, but at least I can ride; at least I can have that blessed time to clear my mind—still one of the most wonderful benefits of bike riding for me.

On this ride, I found myself thinking that almost all my goals for Team Type 1 have or seem to be close to reaching fruition. We've just signed a two-year contract extension with Sanofi-Aventis, the French pharmaceutical giant. We're going to the Giro in 2011 and, it appears ever more likely, to the Tour de France in 2012. So the international dream is coming true.

Sanofi-Aventis and our other big sponsors are investing a ton of money with us—not to promote a specific drug or device but to help communicate the diabetes mission and the message. The same message I've been pounding away at through the years, and in the pages of this book. Take control of your life—you can do it with this disease, in ways that perhaps you couldn't if you had a disease like cancer.

This is a new reality, and it's exciting. Yet, I find a strange inconsistency in my life. Since I was a kid, I've worked hard to control my diabetes, and I've been held up as a role model of control. But when I ran into that old acquaintance at the end of the Twilight race in April 2009 who raised the question of exactly what I was controlling—he was right on the money. What I realized during my meandering ride that afternoon is that Team Type 1 totally controls my life. Everything I do revolves around advancing the team and our mission. I'm proud of it, but I also realize that control of diabetes for the average diabetic should mean something else—the freedom to do other things, the things that people not affected by the disease get to do. In the last couple of years, I've begun to see that I haven't given myself that opportunity. I don't have a personal life; while I do my best to stay in touch with the old crew from Tallahassee, most of my friends are now associated with Team Type 1 or our sponsor organizations. It's all-encompassing and I can't seem to escape from it.

There's an interesting irony here: in the end, diabetes—or specifically my battle against it—*did* end up controlling my life. But only after I'd wrestled the disease to the ground and made it say uncle.

As I've been doing for five years now, I spent a week at Camp Kudzu in the summer of 2010. One of the new campers, a recently diagnosed adolescent girl, came into camp with blood sugar and A1c readings that were very high. Apparently, she was also at Kudzu under duress. "I don't care if I die," she had supposedly told the camp directors.

On the first night of camp, I gave my speech about growing up with diabetes and what I had been able to accomplish as a young adult. This girl was in the audience and I noticed her right away. While most of the kids listened attentively, she sat there, arms crossed, scowling, refusing to make eye contact. She was trying to make it very clear to everyone around her that she did not want to be there. As I related to the kids the condensed version of my childhood and adolescence, told them about my bike racing, RAAM, and Team Type 1, I noticed that she started to perk up. She still wasn't smiling, but she did seem to be paying attention. At the end of the talk, I invited questions, and her hand shot up. *Uh-oh,* I thought. I hoped she wasn't going to make a scene. "I'm glad you became a professional bike rider, and rode across the country and whatever. But have you ever gone to a hospital because of diabetes?"

"Yes," I said, "I had to go several times."

"Really?" she responded, with genuine surprise. "Well . . . how did that make you feel?"

"Hey, it's part of the reality of having type 1. It happens to all of us."

I told her about a few of my blood sugar incidents as a bike racer as well, including the time Daniel Holt may have saved my life in Ireland. She listened intently, and I sensed that maybe this was making an impression.

Later, speaking to her counselor, I found out that she ended up having a great week at Kudzu and seemed to be taking a much more positive, proactive view toward her diabetes. I'm sure it wasn't just my speech that changed her views—Kudzu is such a wonderful, supportive environment—but I think her question, my response, and her subsequent 180-degree turnaround reveal something essential about the challenges facing diabetics, particularly adolescents.

No matter how supportive your family or friends, you feel alone. Heck, I had the most supportive mom in the world, and a neighborhood of people helping us out, but at night I was still the only one who climbed into bed with diabetes. No one else around me could ever really understand what that was like, to be walking around in a seriously malfunctioning body that demanded precise, intense, and constant care—or you could die! And I'd barely known another diabetic until I met Joe. That's probably one reason why I was so determined to prove myself: always focused on me, me, me. That's because you, you, and you didn't have to worry about your blood sugar, and taking injections at certain times, and going blind. *I* was the one with the disease, so why shouldn't I be so fixated on myself?

No doubt, this young lady had struggled with similar issues of isolation, of feeling misunderstood and different—and she was angry about it. Realizing that other diabetics have battled their disease and these emotions, and that we've all had to deal with the consequences—even someone who was being touted as this great bike-riding type 1 "hero"—may have sparked a change in attitude. That night, the light went on for her. I've seen it happen with many others, of all ages. Suddenly, diabetics realize that they *can* take control of it, *can* put diabetes in its place. It could be a type 1, who was born with it, or a type 2, who developed it later. Or it could be a parent who suddenly stops bemoaning the "bad break" that her child has been handed and realizes the positive role that she can and needs to play.

I even believe that the "self-control switch" can illuminate lives that aren't touched by diabetes. It's the change in attitude, for example, that compels somebody who is overweight, who is blaming his or her genes or lack of time or money for not exercising or eating right, to finally get off his butt and out for a walk, to clear out the junk food in the kitchen, and to start taking responsibility for his actions.

Maybe you've already been able to turn on that switch in your life.

If not, what will it take?

I hope that my story will give you a start.

"Strive for 6.5": Plan for Diabetics

Dream Big—all of Team Type 1 did—and won

the Race Across America.

—RAAM BLOG 2007

"What can I do, Phil? What can I do to better control the disease?"

Whether they were kids, parents, or other adults, that's the most common question I hear from diabetics and their families. They're afraid of amputation, blindness, kidney failure. All the worst-case-scenario effects of unchecked diabetes.

I remembered how terrified I was at the prospect of losing my sight. That's when I first starting checking my A1c and using it as a yardstick of my overall diabetes management. It helped me as a kid, which is why later, as the founder of Team Type 1, I came up with the idea of the A1c Challenge.

I discussed it with Dr. Bruce Bode, one of the leading endocrinologists in the country and the medical adviser to many of the major diabetes organizations. I discussed it with those organizations, as well. They wholeheartedly endorsed our program to lower the three-month blood sugar rates to normal levels—or, as we call it, "Strive for 6.5."

The program is relatively simple but addresses the reality of the situation that all of us with type 1 or type 2 deal with.

Diabetes never goes away. It's always there, every mealtime, every day and night. Caring for it is a 365-day-a-year job. So how do you motivate people to rise to the challenge of managing something that's a constant—not to mention an unpleasant and unwanted—part of their lives?

By getting them motivated, challenging them to take the steps they need to and to make the changes in their lives that will help them manage their diabetes, instead of getting overwhelmed by it.

That's why all of us at Team Type 1—riders, management, coaches, bike mechanics—now use "Strive for 6.5" as our signature on e-mails, on the Web sites, and (for the riders), when we sign autographs for kids at the many diabetes camps, conferences, races, and other events we attend. We've gotten hundreds of e-mails from our fans and supporters around the county, telling us about their success in following the Strive for 6.5 Plan.

So if you or someone you love has diabetes, this is my message to you: start now! Team Type 1 *challenges* you to set a goal for your next A1c—to "Strive for 6.5."

First, let's step back for a moment and look at the A1c. This is a commonly used three-month average measure of your blood sugar. The government's National Diabetes Education Program calls the A1c "the best test for you and your health care team to know how well your treatment plan is working over time." We agree—but instead of making it a perfunctory measurement, I recommend using that three-month window as a way to both challenge and reward yourself. The goal is 6.5, which is just a little higher than normal blood sugar, but lower than the 8 or 9 that many diabetics commonly have. While reaching 6.5 doesn't mean your diabetes is "cured," it's something your doctor will applaud, and it shows that you are successfully managing your disease. But it takes work: diet, exercise, determination.

To help motivate you to do that work, and so that this becomes more than "just" a goal of reaching an important but abstract number in a blood test result, let's start by coming up with a reward, a prize you can keep your eye on over the next three months. Maybe it's a vacation for you and your family; a pair of earrings; a special day trip for you and your child. Having that reward in mind will help challenge and motivate you to "Strive for 6.5."

THE A1C "STRIVE FOR 6.5" ACTION PLAN

Figure out your reward. Then think about ways to reward yourself for achieving it. Maybe you'd like a movie night with your friends, or something fun to do with your family? Find something you really want and use that to help stay motivated, positive, and in the moment.

Parents: What is something that your child would want and would make changes to get? A carrot is often just the stimulus needed to get the blood sugars where they need to be. This may be as simple as a night without doing the dishes or seeing a ball game with your child. We are not suggesting bribing your child, but rather that you reward them for their newfound success.

Talk with your physician or diabetes educator before making any drastic changes in your diabetes management. No goal is too high—or too low—as long as your doctor says it's safe.

Next, tell your family and friends about your goal. Explain why it's important to you, and they just may help you stick to the plan.

If you have friends with diabetes, encourage them to take the A1c Challenge with you. Race to see who can get to 6.5 first. A friendly bet always makes competition more exciting.

Now, let's get started on the three-week plan.

Week 1: Out with the Bad!

Eliminate bad habits that lead to what we call "O-o-t"-y ("out-of-target") blood sugars. Pick two or three of these habits and say bye-bye! These habits might include:

- snacking when your blood sugar is high
- eating without checking your blood sugar
- skipping boluses or corrections
- Cutting out candy bars and soft drinks
- Getting down on yourself for a high blood sugar (it happens to the best of us; don't use it as an excuse to quit trying!)

Week 2: In with the Good!

Make three changes that will help your control. Such as:

- *Check more often.* Using your FreeStyle Lite meter four to five *more* times per day can help reduce A1cs up to 3 points. (Team Type 1 founders Phil and Joe check twelve to twenty times per day!) Also, thanks to the rapid result from the FreeStyle Flash, that is only an extra twenty-five seconds per day . . . a small price to pay for eyesight, for example (Phil's motivation).
- *Make more, smaller corrections.* Try a smaller bolus when you're above 150, so that you never get to 200.
- *Eat better.* This week, add one vegetable and one fruit to your diet.

- *Start exercising more often.* You will feel better and achieve better sugar levels.
- *Focus on your fourteen-day average.* Can you lower it 10 points or even 20? Shoot for a fourteen-day average below 130, as this will give you a better overall picture of where your A1c is going.

Check 1.5 hours after bolusing. Testing after you bolus tells you if you took the right amount of insulin and gives you a chance to correct before it's out of range. We are never the same two days in a row, so it never hurts to check it twice!

Week 3: Make it a Habit!

You have now made six changes that will help you to achieve a better A1c. Stick with these practices and they will become habits. Good habits = good (A1c) results.

Don't be shy about what you're doing. Forming habits is a gradual and multifaceted process. Telling more people about what you're doing, and sharing your progress with family, friends, and doctors, is both motivating and reinforcing. So get them onboard.

Moreover, talking about you improvements, no matter how small or gradual ("I haven't had soda in three weeks!") may just push you to want to become even better. Remember that reward at the end, and be patient. It may take six months or nine to get to your goal, but as long as you can get a little better each and every day, then your A1c will continue to improve and you will meet the challenge.

Your A1c already 6.5 or better? What now?

Fantastic! You're in good control. We encourage you to share your story with someone else with diabetes, and help him or her to get there, too. This newfound control will help to empower you to live a better life, and there is no better feeling than helping a friend to keep his eyesight.

Don't Think You Can Do it? Betcha Can!

It may seem difficult to lower your A1c, but I know you can. Consider the example of my Team Type 1 cofounder, Joe Eldridge. When I first met Joe, his A1c was near 11! That's dangerously high. So I challenged Joe to a competition—every time we'd meet, we'd test our sugar levels, and the guy with the higher reading would pay for dinner. For months on end, I ate free and Joe always ended up paying for dinner. Finally, tired of losing, he decided to take the A1c Challenge. His goal was to have me pick up the check for once. He succeeded. Three months later, I was picking up the tab for the burritos, and I know he particularly enjoyed that!

Of course, I was happy to do so. It is worth noting that Joe continues to refine his A1c Challenge. Once he met the Phil-pays-for-dinner goal, he began to set some competitive goals for himself as a rider. Example: Joe's a big guy—he needed to drop some weight to ride at the elite level. That became his A1c Challenge goal. He cut out some junk foods, ramped up his training, and lost forty-five pounds! He is now one of the strongest riders on our team. Joe and I still meet for dinner and still have a friendly A1c competition, but we called a truce. Now we split the dinner bill; in part because, I'm happy to say, we've both met our A1c Challenges, and continue to do so. At this writing, Joe's A1c is 5.6. (Oh, and mine is 5.1, but who's counting?)

THE SWEET TASTE OF 6.5 SUCCESS

Here's an example of how powerful that striving can be. In August 2005, I spoke at a juvenile diabetes camp and urged the kids to do just this: try to lower their blood sugar levels to 6.5 and think about a way to reward themselves when they met that goal. A girl named Lauren, about thirteen, threw the ball back in my court. If she lowered her A1c to 6.5, she said, "what are *you* going to give me?"

For once, I was speechless. I thought about maybe offering her health, well-being, her eyesight, a future. But all I could stammer was, "Well . . . what do you want?"

"Five pounds of candy," she replied.

Again, I hesitated. No diabetic should be gorging on candy, much less a thirteen-year-old, but I wanted her to set the goal of lowering her A1c. Besides, I reasoned, if she made sufficient lifestyle modifications and got her A1c levels well below 6.5, she might be able to have at least some of that candy, anyway. So I took her up on the offer. "Okay, Lauren," I said. "If you meet the Strive for 6.5. goal successfully, I'll buy you five pounds of candy."

Seven months later, I got an e-mail from Lauren, telling me that she had gotten to 6.4. It was time for me to pay up. But, as I read on, I was surprised to see a very specific breakdown of how that five pounds of candy was to be remitted: "My mom wants white chocolate, my dad wants dark chocolate, my brother wants Skittles, and my sister wants Starbursts."

This wasn't for her! It was for her family, who, as an act of solidarity with Lauren, had all eschewed sweets. So the reward she wanted was really a reward for them. I was deeply moved by this act of selflessness. It's a reminder to all of us with diabetes that we owe a great deal of gratitude to those around us who have supported and helped us. Short of a few pounds of chocolates, I think the best way to thank them is to double our resolve to fight and manage this disease, to do the things necessary to keep us healthy. That's the ultimate challenge and the ultimate reward—to the people you love and to yourself.

You can do it—you can manage your diabetes and live a full, active, and healthy life—and the A1c Challenge is the way to start! So let's go for a ride to a future where you are in control of your diabetes.

I know you will enjoy the rewards.

LESSONS LEARNED FROM A CRACK SHOT

You can think of diabetes management as trying to hit a moving target—and I am a crack shot.

I've devoted my life to becoming an expert diabetes "marksman," to striking the balance between blood sugar that's popping or crashing. If a physician tested my blood sugar right now, he or she wouldn't even know I was diabetic. I got good at it by monitoring my body constantly, training hard, and eating right. Part of my obsession over this is because I view myself as a role model to others with type 1. I want to show other diabetics that it can be done. They just have to put some effort into it. I've told you about A1c. Here are a couple of other tips I've learned that can help make things easier for you or your family.

For parents of children with type 1 diabetes: how to make Halloween a really sweet holiday for your child

Halloween can be a difficult time for a diabetic. Eating a lot of candy and other sweets is out, so there's a tendency for concerned parents to want to keep their children from trick-or-treating. The result is that they feel labeled as a kid with a disease. When I was a kid, my mom was concerned that I would feel ostracized during Halloween. She knew I couldn't be wolfing down candy, but she didn't want me to sit home while all my friends were out trick-or-treating. So she came up with a wonderful way for me to enjoy Halloween. You can do the same thing I did:

Every Halloween, we'd dress up in our Power Ranger or Batman costumes and go out trick-or-treating in our Tallahassee neighborhood. At the end of the day, my buddies would give me whatever candy they didn't want. I would take this massive pile of candy—what I had collected and what my friends had given me—and I would sell it back to my mom. She paid twenty-five cents for chocolate and ten cents for anything else. That was her idea and it worked. Halloween became one of my favorite days of the year: we'd spend a lot of time, and my mom knew she didn't have to worry about my feeling left out or stigmatized. And I made a profit! So, for this Halloween, make a sweet deal with your child!

For adults battling type 1 diabetes: choose your "Magnificent Seven"

When I was a kid, my mom gave a crash course in diabetes education and management to everyone on our block, every one of my friends and their parents, everyone in my school. Now, Joanna Southerland is a thorough and determined woman. While you may not have to run clinics for your neighborhood, you do need to make sure that key people in your life are aware of what they need to do just in case you should have what we call a "hypo"—a life-threatening episode of hypoglycemic shock.

Now that I don't have my mom running around educating people on my behalf, I make a point to tell everyone that I like and think I might hang out or spend some time with, "If I start acting dumber than normal, make me drink a soda or a sugared sports drink, and then have me test my blood sugar. And if I pass out, you dial 911." That took the edge of concern off for me. My friends learned a little bit and, I hoped, would be ready to respond.

Some people have trouble discussing something so personal with people they really don't know that well, yet. And granted, confiding in people you've just met can be a risky thing. Also, there are some people who may not want the responsibility, which can make for an awkward situation. So if you're not comfortable with discussing a "hypo" with the guy you just met at the gym, or everybody in the cubicles adjacent to yours on the new job, or your entire night-school class, well then, think about *seven*—that's seven key people in your life, at least one of whom you're likely to be around on a day-to-day basis. Try to choose at least one from every aspect of your life: at least one family member, one friend that you socialize with, one co-worker, one neighbor, and maybe one person likely to be present at and involved with the major activities of your life (so, one person from your church, one person on your softball team, and so on).

These are your Magnificent Seven. Explain your disease to them; teach them what to do if and when you ever have a "hypo."

Oh yeah—and treat 'em nicely. Every one of my Magnificent Seven—most of whom have been around me for a long time—has probably helped saved my life at one point or another.

Those seven are some of the first people my coauthor and I want to thank.

An Open Letter: Twenty-eight Years Later

Dear Mom and Dad,

I know you both just got the news that if I were to live to twenty-five, I would most likely be blind.

However, I want you to know that it is going to be okay. You are going to push me into the world knowing that, with the exception of a few insulin injections a day, I am the same as every other kid in the world. You are going to teach me the value of exercise and hard work, and you are going to enable me to live. I would like to ask you to do a few things for me and give you a few tips on this little game we call diabetes.

I want you to know first and foremost, that this is not your fault. Diabetes is something I now consider to be a gift, and it is perhaps the greatest one you ever gave me (aside from my first bike). We don't choose diabetes, rather diabetes chooses those who can handle it.

Please learn everything you can on this disease. Knowledge is power and your thirst for information in the early years will make my life and my habits much better in the years to come. Please don't ever take it easy on me because I have this disease. I am not different, I just have to make adjustments. I also want you to know that whatever technology you currently are using to control my blood sugar is going to change, and will change drastically. At first it will be overwhelming, but it will get better and better. The technology is going to point out our errors. I am going to have high blood sugars and will go to the hospital because of them, and I am going to have low blood sugars, which will also take me to the hospital. But I will live!

Mom, you are going to watch me have seizures, and please know that even though I will come to the brink of death on more than a few occasions, it's not my time yet, and more importantly, it's not your fault. I am a fighter, Mom, and that is how you have raised me. You will do things for me that will help to revolutionize the world of diabetes, and I promise that one day you will be able to sleep through the night. I would like to ask you to do one thing for the family, and that is for any amount of attention you give to me as a diabetic kid, please give equal or more attention to my brother (yes, you will have another) as he grows up. The odd thing is that in a family of a kid with diabetes, the sibling without diabetes is often "the othered."

I am going to fight with you, and I am going to argue. I will even refuse to eat broccoli. But I ask that you sit there with me for two hours until I finally cave and eat it. Your stubbornness will define my being for the better, and I will try to take all the good that you are, and the heart and soul you put into me, and pass it on to the children of the world. Please let me know the side effects that poor control and discipline can bring. Please don't let me take for granted the fact that I have insulin and test strips. I feel extremely lucky for the people that you will bring into our lives, and for the lessons you will enable me to learn.

In hindsight, I would also like to thank you for standing strong when I argued about college. Your decision for me to go was brilliant, as was your "business plan" call several years later. As time will tell, you have been right about a lot. You have done this because if you believe it to be a lie, then it is a lie, or if you believe it to be true, then it is true.

This is the very same belief system and passion that you have instilled upon me. It is because of everything that you have done that I now see it as wrong that children do not have access to the supplies I once tried to refuse taking. It is because of this that I will not quit working until they have them in their hands, and they know how to use them.

I know I may sometimes seem distant and unavailable, and for that I am sorry. I am sorry I don't call or write like a "normal son" does, or that I only come home once per year now. You have instilled in me "The Power to Change" and with that power comes responsibility. Just as you once gave up everything to ensure I stayed alive, I too now give up some things to ensure these other kids live. I have a dream now, Mom, a dream that I wake up in a world where nobody goes blind from diabetes. It is your commitment toward ensuring that I can still see (which I can) that will one day ensure we all see.

Mom, Dad, Jack (yes, you will name my brother Jack): I love you all. You are my family and have been there when I truly needed you, and am forever grateful for your love and support. You are in a dire time right now, but again I would like you to know that I have many years left in me, and I hope you raise me just the same in this second round. It's still not my time!

Love and thanks,
Philpott

Index